Cancer Is
Complicated

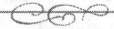

Cancer Is Complicated

AND OTHER UNEXPECTED LESSONS I'VE LEARNED

Clea Shearer

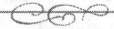

THE OPEN FIELD / PENGUIN LIFE

VIKING
An imprint of Penguin Random House LLC
1745 Broadway, New York, NY 10019
penguinrandomhouse.com

The Open Field/A Penguin Life Book

THE OPEN FIELD is a registered
trademark of MOS Enterprises, Inc.

VIKING is a registered trademark of Penguin Random House LLC.

Designed by Alexis Sulaimani

LIBRARY OF CONGRESS CONTROL NUMBER: 2024059685
ISBN 9780593830611 (hardcover)
ISBN 9780593830628 (ebook)

Printed in the United States of America
1st Printing

The authorized representative in the EU for product
safety and compliance is Penguin Random House Ireland,
Morrison Chambers, 32 Nassau Street, Dublin D02 YH68,
Ireland, https://eu-contact.penguin.ie.

MARIA SHRIVER

PRESENTS

THE OPEN FIELD

A PUBLISHING IMPRINT

BOOKS THAT RISE ABOVE THE NOISE AND MOVE HUMANITY FORWARD

Dear Reader,

Years ago, these words attributed to Rumi found a place in my heart:

> *Out beyond ideas of*
> *wrongdoing and rightdoing,*
> *there is a field. I'll meet you there.*

Ever since, I've cultivated an image of what I call "the Open Field"—a place out beyond fear and shame, beyond judgment, loneliness, and expectation. A place that hosts the reunion of all creation. It's the hope of my soul to find my way there—and whenever I hear an insight or a practice that helps me on the path, I love nothing more than to share it with others.

That's why I've created The Open Field. My hope is to publish books that honor the most unifying truth in human life: We are all seeking the same things. We're all seeking dignity. We're all seeking joy. We're all seeking love and acceptance, seeking to be seen, to be safe. And there is no competition for these things we seek—because they are not material goods; they are spiritual gifts!

We can all give each other these gifts if we share what we know—what has lifted us up and moved us forward. That is our duty to one another—to help each other toward acceptance, toward peace, toward happiness—and my promise to you is that the books published under this imprint will be maps to the Open Field, written by guides who know the path and want to share it.

Each title will offer insights, inspiration, and guidance for moving beyond the fears, the judgments, and the masks we all wear. And when we take off the masks, guess what? We will see that we are the opposite of what we thought— we are each other.

We are all on our way to the Open Field. We are all helping one another along the path. I'll meet you there.

Love, Maria S

For my mother, who gave me strength, courage, and love.
I wouldn't be here without you, in more ways than one.

Contents

*Cancer Is
Complicated*

Everyone Says It's a Journey but No One Says Where You're Going

If you're the type of person who likes having control over a situation, cancer is not the disease for you. The organizer in me had a hard time understanding how quickly things could change, hour by hour, day by day. Whether I liked it or not (I did not like it), I had to relinquish my desire to manage the process, and trust the process instead.

This book is called *Cancer Is Complicated* because my journey has ranged from uncomfortable to comforting, unbearable to doable, isolated to embraced, and scared to confident. Cancer is not just one thing or one experience. It's layered, and nuanced, and *certainly* full of surprises. Above all, it's not linear. It's called a journey for a reason. There isn't really a beginning or an end, but we take the ups with the downs, the wins with the losses, and we fight like hell the entire time.

Before I dive into my story, I should give you a little background on who I am.

My name is Clea Shearer (hi!), and I'm best known for cofounding a company called The Home Edit with my best friend, Joanna

Teplin. We started our business as strictly in-home professional organizers, just the two of us. That business evolved to multiple team members across multiple cities, social platforms with millions of followers, three *New York Times* bestselling books, a Netflix show, and a line of organizing products in countries all over the world.

In August 2015, Joanna and I began building this business like it was a child we were raising together, and we took no breaks from the work. Speaking of children, I also have two of them, and they are not business-related: my daughter, Stella Blue, and my son, Sutton Gray. I would have none of the above without my husband, John Shearer. He will come up quite a few times in this book, and for good reason, because he gets tens across the board.

Way back in the summer of 2021, Joanna and I were asked by Netflix to appear on a ridiculous show called *Floor Is Lava*, a giant version of the kids' game in which you have to navigate an obstacle course and fly through the air on a makeshift trapeze to avoid falling into the "lava," which in this case was a viscous slime the consistency of honey.

We, along with other reality-show personalities, would compete to see who could stay out of the goo the longest. Spoiler: It wasn't me. While trying to jump from one piece of floating fake furniture to another, I wiped out and went under. I had to throw out my clothes and take three showers in the studio before leaving the set. But I also had to get into the shower as soon as I got to the hotel to keep scrubbing. As I lathered up, I felt something on my right breast. Or did I?

I wondered for a second if it could possibly be . . . but no, of course, it couldn't. I was just being paranoid. It didn't hurt, and it wasn't a big lump or anything. Breasts are lumpy in general, and I tend to be an overthinker. To counteract that, I said to myself, *Clea, stop it. You're fine.* Then I went back to removing the weird honey slime and forgot about it almost entirely.

Back then, I didn't understand how fast cancer can grow, and how little decisions like dismissing what feels like a lump rather than seeing a doctor right away can dramatically change an outcome. We all know how prevalent breast cancer is, and the stats that come along with it: One in eight women will be diagnosed at some point in their lifetime. But what I came to learn is how quickly the course of your life can change forever by not taking every preventive measure possible.

Looking back, I don't want to believe that I was feeling a tumor that day in the shower. Because that would mean I could have gotten screened in July 2021, and maybe most of what followed could have been avoided. But I can't dwell in regret, and I can't consume myself with questions that can't be answered. All I can do is focus my energy on telling you what happened to me, in the hope that it resonates.

Some of you might have just been diagnosed. Some of you might be in treatment. Some of you might be survivors. And some of you might be partners, friends, or loved ones trying to understand the path ahead. However all of us got here, we're in a club we never asked to be a part of.

If you've received a diagnosis, I hope hearing my account will provide some companionship and solace as you navigate this new reality. If you have a loved one dealing with the disease, I hope this will give you a sense of what they're going through, and the best ways to help.

And to those who cancer hasn't yet touched, I hope this book will give you a sense of what so much of the world is dealing with at any given time.

The good news is that a few months ago I rang THE BELL, the symbolic end to cancer treatment. I want to acknowledge that not everyone *gets* to ring the bell, because for some, cancer treatment never ends. If you are fortunate enough to commemorate the end like I was, ring the bell for everyone around you too. It is not lost on me that I am one of the lucky ones. I received excellent medical care, and it worked. But make no mistake, I am still *very much* affected by this disease. It's taken a permanent toll on my body, and in some ways it's completely remade my identity. Living with cancer isn't something I would recommend, but in some ways, it's changed me for the better and taught me lessons I otherwise never would have learned.

One Thing

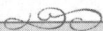

This book focuses on my experience with breast cancer, but I hope my story will prove useful to people dealing with all types of cancer. Many cancers will involve treatment via surgery and some combination of chemotherapy and radiation, or one or the other. Sometimes doctors may offer you chemotherapy via pills. Oral chemotherapy might be given in addition to or even instead of an IV in certain circumstances. Other types of treatment might include receiving a stem cell or bone marrow transplant, or immunotherapy. What I hope everyone can relate to through my own account of having cancer is that this journey encompasses a lot of twists and turns through hills and valleys. There are physical discomforts and pain, mental anguish, and fears and worries—yet at the same time you might have stronger relationships, find humor and beauty in small things, or have a new perspective on life. You will almost definitely discover that you are much braver than you ever gave yourself credit for.

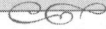

CHAPTER ONE

Cancer Doesn't Care If You're Busy

It's not that easy to detect breast cancer unless you know what you're looking for. You have to be in touch with your body to know when something is not normal. Otherwise, you might end up like me. I ignored the lump I felt in July 2021 and wrote it off, sure that nothing was wrong.

The number of things that I worry about, especially since COVID, make me hyperalert all the time. I am essentially a meerkat. But I didn't actually think *I could have cancer.* No way. There was no probability of it in my mind, nothing so severe. It was an impossibility. So, I moved through my life as usual.

And I had to say, life was really good. Joanna and I had a wonderful summer filming the second season of our show, *Get Organized with The Home Edit*, and then started a lot of exciting projects. Everything was firing on all cylinders through the end of 2021. It was the best of times, truly. That fall, in October, I went to Paris with my mother, her best friend, Sherry, and Sherry's daughter, Merritt, who's one of *my* best friends, for a girls' trip after filming wrapped.

The trip to Paris was one of the happiest moments of my life, one of the highest highs, even though we were all so nervous with another COVID wave happening. Merritt has multiple sclerosis and she's immunocompromised, plus our moms are in their seventies, which puts them at high risk. I was the only one who was seemingly healthy, saying things like, "I'll take one for the team and touch the doorknob!"

After Paris I got back to work, jet-setting with Joanna to multiple cities, attending meetings around the clock, speaking at events, launching new products. Most important, that December, The Home Edit started the process of being acquired by Hello Sunshine, Reese Witherspoon's media company. To say this was a dream come true would be dramatically underselling the situation. In fact, who has dreams like this? Even my dreams have limits. It was very, very big. We couldn't contain our excitement.

So it was no surprise that in 2022 I started thinking: *This is going to be the best year of my life.* I was on cloud nine, and I was going to celebrate. I was turning forty on February 1, and I decided to throw myself an over-the-top birthday party for the first time ever. I honestly kind of hate throwing parties, because at my core, I am still insecure and nervous people won't come, or that something will go wrong, and there are too many unpredictable outcomes to consider. I'm getting anxious just thinking about it. But I decided to go for it and threw a party I'll never forget.

The room was filled to the brim with candles and rainbow flowers, and so many of our friends in Nashville, where my family and I live, came out for the night. Some even grabbed the mic to perform, which was pretty magical. It was definitely a night to remember, and I'm so glad I have that memory.

On February 18, 2022, Joanna and I announced to our team that we were being acquired by Hello Sunshine. We had had to keep it a secret up until then, for a few months, until the contracts were fully executed. We invited everyone in Nashville to come to the office, and we had a big TV screen with all our other employees Zooming in from throughout the country. And then . . . Reese walked into the room, under a rainbow arch of balloons, and welcomed us all to the Hello Sunshine family.

It was the proudest moment of my life, and an incredible experience that I will never, ever forget. A few days later, we were flying to New York to do press for all the exciting things we had in the works for the company, like the new season of *Get Organized* (which was scheduled to premiere April 1), and the launch of our first magazine. Everything felt electric. Perfect, even. It's funny because I've always been superstitious about things being perfect. Nothing can be *that* good without there being a glitch.

And then came February 22. Joanna and I were still in New York and had a bunch of press lined up that day. As I washed up in the shower that morning, I distinctly felt a lump—possibly even two lumps—in my right breast. Nothing ambiguous about it this time.

One Thing

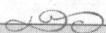

How to Do a Breast Self-Exam

According to Mount Sinai Health System, you should give yourself a breast self-exam once a month. Here is some more information from them about how to conduct a monthly breast self-exam:

The best day to do a self-exam is three to five days after your period ends. Your breasts are naturally less lumpy right after your period, so there's less chance that you'll mistake a normal bump for an abnormal growth. If you've already gone through menopause and your periods have stopped, just do your exam on the same day every month. Mark it on your calendar so you won't forget. To do the exam, lie on your back, as it's easier to feel any lumps or changes when you're lying down. First, put your right hand behind your head. Then, using the middle fingers on your left hand, gently but firmly press down, circling your entire breast. Make sure you cover the whole right breast. Squeeze your nipple gently. See if any fluid comes out. Now sit up, and feel around your armpit. When you're done with the right breast, repeat the whole check on the left side. Next, stand in front of a mirror. With your arms down at your sides, look at both breasts. Check the shape of each breast. Look for any changes in the skin, like dimpling or puckering. Also see if your nipples have become inverted. Now do the same check with your arms over your head. After you've done a few breast self-exams, you'll become familiar with the look and shape of your breasts. At each exam, you're looking for anything different, like new bumps, changes in the texture of your skin, or discharge from your nipples. If you do notice that something has changed, don't panic, it could mean many different things. But call your doctor as soon as you can so you can find out what's caused the change and, if necessary, get it treated.

In a routine breast exam, or even a quick rinse in the shower, you might come across a lump that feels new. Some might be nothing, and some might be something, but only your doctor can make that determination. If you're on the fence about whether to act, jump off the fence and pick up the phone.

Additional Resources for How to Do a Breast Self-Exam

keep-a-breast.org or the Keep a Breast app

breastcancer.org

mayoclinic.org

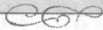

CHAPTER TWO

The Realization

For a brief moment, even when I felt the lump, I still thought, *There's no way this is that kind of lump. There's just no way that this could be happening to me. No way that this is cancer.* But then one second later I thought, *Well . . . why isn't it cancer and why couldn't it be happening to me?*

When I thought about it that way, there was actually *no* reason it wouldn't be cancer, no logic behind why I would be exempt. I think what I meant was: I didn't *want* it to be me; this simply wasn't ever in my future plans. This was meant to be the highest point of my life, and cancer couldn't get in the way of that. Except that it absolutely could, and maybe it would.

I tried to make a list of all the millions of things it could be. A blocked milk duct? People definitely get those. Sure, it had been years since I had breastfed a baby, but maybe it was residual. That felt like a stretch. Maybe it was something totally benign—a cyst? My mind was racing in the shower, going over every possibility I could think of. And then it just hit me like a ton of bricks. There wasn't another possibility. It was a lump. It was the kind of lump that people are talking about when they say, "I found a lump." This was the lump.

I didn't rule out the possibility of it still being something else, but it was undeniably a lump—a very large lump or potentially even two lumps. I was scared to even get out of the shower and confront this reality.

As I had just turned forty only three weeks earlier, I was due for my first mammogram. I was going to have to start thinking about my breast health. It all started to click in my brain that I needed to call the doctor *immediately.*

By the time I stepped out of the shower and dried off, I was shaking, trying to unlock my mobile phone so I could call my gynecologist. Part of me was speechless, thinking, *I can't believe I'm about to say these words.*

The receptionist picked up. "Hello, office of [someone I will not name]," she said.

"Hi, this is Clea Shearer," I said, the way I had so many times before. "I need to schedule my well-woman appointment, but I also need to schedule my first mammogram. I am pretty sure I just found a lump. . . ."

My words hung dry in my throat; I was still in disbelief that they needed to come out of my mouth. *I found a lump.* Meanwhile, my mind had no problem screaming, *This is an emergency!*

This was very different from calling the doctor for an annual appointment, a checkup or wellness exam. If you say that you have something wrong right now, they tend to prioritize your situation because it's urgent. I wasn't asking to do something *preventive.* I needed care *right now.* But that didn't even seem to matter in this case.

"I'm sorry," the receptionist said, "but there are no appointments available on the books with the doctor. We're completely booked through April, and the May books aren't open yet, so we can't put you on the schedule at this time. Try back sometime next month to see if the May calendar is open."

"You're telling me you can't even schedule me for May?" I said. "It's February. There's no appointment currently available and no appointment that you're able to book even after that?"

"That's correct," she said.

"How is this allowed in health care? I am telling you I have something potentially cancerous in my body and you're not able to fit me in?" I was truly shocked and outraged. "I can't even get a mammogram?"

"No, unfortunately not."

I was still scared, but now I was also livid. How in the world was it possible that I was not able to get an appointment? There I was, telling this receptionist that I'd found a lump in my breast. Doesn't "I feel a lump" set off a breast cancer bat signal of some sort? Surely someone would be able to see me to get this sorted out. Why on earth wouldn't they escalate this beyond what appointments they had available?

Inaction on their part would normally trigger a response of, *Well, I suppose I'll just have to wait for a mammogram. I guess I'll just have to make an appointment whenever I'm able to get an appointment.* No one loves going to the doctor, so when they tell you they can fit you in months later, you just take it and are semi-grateful you can put it off for a while. Sometimes I call the dentist and they say nothing's available until whatever faraway date. I silently say thank you and then tell them I'll be there. But this time, my gut was telling me—screaming at me—that I had to fight this one out.

I could postpone getting it looked at, but I just knew that I had already waited too long. Alternatively, I could find a way to get seen and not take no for an answer.

I am so, so grateful that I listened to my instincts and didn't take the complacent option for once. That I didn't sit back and say, *Well, I guess I just have to wait awhile. What's a few months?* I decided instead of waiting to possibly get an appointment in May, I would be relentless until I exhausted all my options.

Within minutes, I called my excellent primary care physician, Dr. Kurtz, at Vanderbilt Health, in a panic. And to my relief, she responded the way I hoped she would: "As soon as you're back in Nashville, we're going to get you in for a mammogram and an ultrasound. We need to get this checked immediately."

I was so thankful to have someone in my corner. Of course, I was scared for these tests and what they might confirm, but I realized knowing was better than not, and I went ahead and scheduled the appointments. Thank goodness my doctor heard me, listened to me, and activated all channels to make it happen.

Dr. Kurtz was the first person I told about my lump (with the exception of the receptionist at the other doctor's office), but the next phone call was going to be much harder. How on earth could I tell my husband something this major over the phone? I didn't give myself time to consider the question, because with every second that passed, I felt like I was keeping a secret from him. I also didn't give myself enough time to consider how I was going to approach this conversation, and once John answered the phone, I came in hot in full panic mode. John is very levelheaded and calm, so he reminded me that just because I had felt something didn't mean it was definitely cancer. We would let the scans speak for themselves and try not to get ahead of ourselves.

After New York, Joanna and I were scheduled to be in Houston to meet with one of our retailers at a huge conference. The dates were set in stone, so I planned my mammogram and ultrasound appointment in Nashville for the following week. While we were at the hotel in Houston, I asked Joanna to feel my breast. I needed her gut reaction. I wanted to know if she was thinking the same thing I was thinking.

My lump was large enough to feel through my shirt; I didn't even need to pull it up. She looked up at me and said, "Okay, I definitely feel what you're talking about, but that does not mean that it's cancer. It's definitely something, but it's not necessarily cancer. It could be a million other things." She paused. "I'm glad you're getting this checked out, though, because I think you need to."

"Okay," I said, "that's right."

In some ways I felt validated that I wasn't being overdramatic. In other ways I thought, *Well, here we go.* In that moment, I just knew. I didn't even need medical confirmation; I was just certain as we left Houston to return to Nashville: *I have breast cancer.*

One Thing

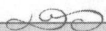

You are your best advocate—especially when it comes to your health. Even if you're not a medical expert, you *are* an expert in knowing how your body feels. If you suspect something is wrong, do not take no for an answer. Speak up, insist on receiving care, and if you reach a dead end, find an alternative option.

If advocating for yourself is something you struggle with, Deb Gordon, the author of *The Health Care Consumer's Manifesto*, suggests that you pretend you're advocating for someone you love. She writes:

> What would you do if you felt your mother or your best friend were getting the run-around in their health care encounters? Or if your child's doctor was not paying attention to their symptoms?
>
> Chances are, you'd stomp up and down—metaphorically anyway—and insist that they get more attention. You might counsel a friend to speak up or get a second opinion. You might feel scared of the impact of a missed diagnosis, and angry if something bad happened because they didn't advocate for themselves.
>
> When it comes to your own health concerns, you are the mom, the child, or the best friend to those people who care about you. Don't you owe it to them to follow your own advice?

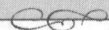

CHAPTER THREE

What's Going On?

My time at the Houston airport waiting for my flight back to Nashville was mostly spent sobbing in a restaurant booth while drinking whatever wine they had at the bar. The very real possibility that I was sick was starting to sink in, and I was caught between whether to believe it or tell myself there was still *no way*. Joanna, who was sitting with me at the airport, was leaning toward the no-way camp, but I could see the fear in her eyes. We both agreed, however, that we needed confirmation before fully unraveling.

My mammogram and ultrasound appointment wasn't for a few more days, so I did the only proactive thing I could think of: I started to put together a plan, take notes, and gather information. I immediately called a few key people in my life. Merritt, who I mentioned previously, is not just one of my best friends; she's family. If anyone could help me wrap my head around a life-altering disease, it was going to be her. Then I started calling my close friends who are breast cancer survivors.

One was Christina Applegate. She has been my close friend for a long time, but she has been a breast cancer warrior and health advocate even longer. *No one* tells you the truth like Christina. She answered every single one of my questions and somehow gave me the space to cry, the ability to laugh, and important perspective. Next, I called my friend Lauren R., who did the same. And I called my friend Stevie. To hear their voices, knowing they had once been in this position too, filled me with deep comfort. And also sadness, because of just *how many* of us have found ourselves experiencing the same thing.

I was desperate for any information I could get my hands on. What does a tumor feel like? How big is big? Is it normal to be able to feel something through my clothing? What if it *is* cancer—what happens next? Will it hurt? I didn't have a formal list of questions to ask, so everything just tumbled out of my mouth in rapid succession. I knew there would be a million more phone calls like this, and each one would surely provide the same amount of honesty, tears, and comfort all rolled into one conversation.

As I made these calls and said the words out loud, "I think I have breast cancer," it shook me to my core. It felt like a possibility that was turning into a probability. Every time I said the words, it became even more real. I was worried that I was somehow willing the reality into existence by even having these conversations.

Once I got home, I walked over to John in the kitchen and blurted out, "I feel like it's definitely breast cancer."

"No, I really don't think so. It could be a million things," he said. "We're going to go get you screened and they're going to tell you that it's something you don't have to worry about. And it will be good to have that peace of mind before we leave for spring break."

Before I'd found the lump, John and I had planned to fly to

California over spring break with the kids. We were going to spend a week there visiting John's mom, and then John and I would leave the kids with his mom and go on to Paris for a romantic vacation, just the two of us.

"Well, I hope you're right," I said, but honestly, I was losing faith that it was going to be anything other than a confirmation of my worst fear.

I'd felt my lump on February 22, 2022, and now it was March 8. Finally, it was time for my mammogram and bilateral ultrasound appointment. John came with me.

He and I arrived nervously gripping each other's hands. I asked if he was able to come back with me, but he was told he had to wait in the lobby because male visitors were not allowed farther into the breast center. The nurse had warned us that the back-to-back procedures might take a while, so he got comfortable, and I headed back to get started. I knew he was still thinking I was going to be in and out with a clean bill of health. But in my gut, I knew this appointment wasn't going to pan out that way.

Without John, I felt a little intimidated. I was given a robe—not a gown, just a waffled bathrobe that said Vanderbilt Breast Center on the chest—and pointed toward a bathroom where I could change. I started to panic a little. As I put on my bathrobe, I took a quick selfie because it was International Women's Day and I wanted to encourage other women to get their mammograms too. I didn't realize that I was taking the picture I would later use to announce my cancer diagnosis.

After I left the bathroom, I entered an interior waiting room full of women of all ages, all waiting for the same appointment. I wondered, *Are all these women here for routine mammograms? Or did anyone else in this room come in because they felt a lump? Are other people in this room afraid, or are they here for prevention?*

I didn't know the circumstances for everyone around me and why they were there, but I was curious if anyone's situation was similar to mine. Some were laughing and making jokes while commenting on the home improvement show on TV. I figured that group probably wasn't worried, and I was jealous of how carefree they appeared. Then there were the people who were fairly somber, and I wondered if they already knew . . . or if, like me, they thought they knew.

I'd never been in a communal waiting room like this before, where clearly we were all there for similar reasons but would leave with very different outcomes. While I sat there, I wondered how each of us would leave the office. Some were surely going to go home to their families without a second thought, and some would have to sit in the parking lot processing next steps. This was a breast clinic, and one in eight women get breast cancer. There were more than eight people in the room, so it wasn't hard to do the math. Would I be the one, or among the lucky seven?

Eventually, they called me back for my mammogram.

But before I continue, let me pause to tell you what a mammogram is actually like, in case you haven't had one.

You will surely hear that mammograms are the worst. Some women say they range from uncomfortable to downright painful. Mammograms need better PR! They can, without question, be painful for some people. But overall, they are totally fine. Do I want to get one for fun on a Saturday? No. But we all need to stop being afraid of mammograms because they are *not* a torture instrument. Now, the news mammograms might provide *is* worth worrying about. But putting off any potential bad news only creates a worse situation.

Okay, moving on from my PSA . . . My mammogram started with my left breast. This part was not nerve-racking because I knew my right breast was the issue. My left breast was totally fine. So, as we went through all the motions, I had anxious butterflies in my stomach about the right breast coming up next.

Once my right breast was being scanned, I couldn't stop myself from asking the technician, "What do you see? Can you see something? Can you tell if anything is wrong?"

You probably won't be surprised to hear that the technicians will not tell you *anything*. That's not their job. I totally get it, but it wasn't going to stop me from *trying* to get my tech to share what she knew. I wondered if she could immediately tell what the lump was. She had to have an inkling, right? I was dying to get even the bare minimum of information. I would be happy with an educated guess at this point.

We did a variety of angles, on all sides: sitting, standing, leaning. It was thorough. I assumed my mammogram was standard practice, but it was my first, so what did I know? If they had asked me to hop on one foot and cluck like a chicken, I would have done it.

Afterward, I felt anxious, but relatively okay. I thought, *If it was cancer, wouldn't alarm bells be going off? Isn't there a red phone that would start to ring and everyone would come rushing in?* The nurse certainly wasn't looking at me with sad eyes. She was not giving me any signals that would indicate she knew or was thinking this was a serious situation. So, I felt momentarily hopeful reading the tea leaves.

I was then shuffled from the mammogram room to the ultrasound room. I hoisted myself onto the bed, and I felt the cool gel placed on my chest and the prodding exam tool—very reminiscent of a pregnancy exam. I looked up at the screen and could see they were isolating two masses that were lit up in color. I don't know why I consider myself a radiologist in moments like this. Why even bother trying to decipher what anything means when I went to art school? But there was a lot of pointing and murmuring, and I could see out of the corner of my eye that the ultrasound tech had just brought in someone else in a white coat. That couldn't be good.

The new person introduced herself as the radiologist who was going to take a look at the ultrasound and give a recommendation about next steps. As the team started discussing my case in hushed voices, I couldn't help but ask, "Is it bad? Is there something bad?"

"I cannot say for certain," the radiologist said, "but the growths are cause for significant concern, and should be biopsied immediately."

"Do you think it's cancer?" I asked.

She repeated that she could not say for certain. "I cannot make that determination. Only a biopsy can tell us that information." I explained that I was actually leaving for California the next day, and then Paris, so I couldn't get a biopsy until I returned in a few weeks. She paused and said, "You can't leave the country without getting a biopsy. In fact, I don't want you leaving this building without getting this biopsied." And with that, she left the room to try to secure an appointment for me that evening. Which left me on my own to absolutely spiral.

At this point, John had been out in the waiting room for hours, but I hadn't had a chance to look at my phone. He had texted me, *Any news, any updates?*

I didn't know what to say. All I could text back was, *It's not good news.*

Of course, that wasn't helpful, but I didn't know how else to describe the situation. Was it definitely *bad* news? No one had said that. The radiologist would have told me if anything had been definitive. She wasn't leaving me hanging, she just genuinely didn't know the answer. Right?

They want to do a biopsy right away, I finally wrote back. *Like within the hour.*

By this point it was late in the day and I was starting to get texts from my mother and Joanna, both of whom knew I was going in for my scans today. They assumed I had finished much earlier and that no news was good news. I called my mother from the ultrasound room while I was waiting for further instructions. The second I heard her voice I started sobbing and couldn't catch my breath. Instinctively, she started sobbing too, even though no words were said. We didn't even have to speak. She knew exactly what I was telling her. I remember her saying words of disbelief and asking a couple of questions, but it was honestly a blur. I had to hang up quickly because the radiologist had entered the room again.

I was still crying uncontrollably when she said they had managed to fit me into the schedule. Why wasn't she comforting me and telling me this was just standard? Why wasn't she telling me there was a good chance I would be totally fine? I was starting to read between the lines; any hope I had left was starting to evaporate. Through a haze, I remember being told I would be getting a triple biopsy on both potential tumors and surrounding lymph nodes to see if whatever it was had spread.

I could barely see straight through my tears, but I had an hour before my next appointment, so I put on my clothes and headed toward the lobby to see John.

One Thing

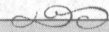

Mammograms are relatively painless, but cancer isn't. Getting checked could not only save your life but also prevent the difficulty of surgery and treatment. Not *knowing* you have cancer isn't the same thing as not *having* cancer.

There are free and low-cost mammograms available if you aren't insured. Organizations such as Susan G. Komen and the American Cancer Society can help you find them. There are also plenty of free or low-cost options available at imaging centers during October, Breast Cancer Awareness Month.

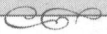

CHAPTER FOUR

The Biopsy

I walked through the doors to the lobby, and the second I saw John with tears on his face, I crumpled into a ball. Neither of us had words yet, and even if we did, I think we were far too afraid to say them out loud.

We walked out of the building clutching each other's hands and got in his car to collect ourselves. I repeated everything I could remember, and how ominous the exam room had felt. I had never had a medical experience like this before. Usually there is a suggestion of it possibly being this, or maybe being that. But while no one would tell me anything definitive, there were nothing but definitive looks in their eyes.

I needed to talk to someone who could give me a better idea of what was happening. Dr. Kurtz had been the one to set up these appointments, and she was able to see all the results in real time. I got in touch to ask if she could talk and she called me in about thirty seconds. When I answered the phone, I was—you guessed it—crying. My inability to form sentences and only sob was quickly becoming a pattern.

"Try to remain calm," she told me. "Don't panic."

But as the conversation continued, I realized that she was moving directly into planning mode. She was using gentle language, but it was very clear that she believed the biopsy would confirm these were cancerous tumors, and preparing for that outcome was the most pragmatic approach.

"I have the most incredible colleagues in oncology who I would love to introduce you to, should you need it," she said. I could tell I was going to need it.

I could barely take in the information because I was practically hyperventilating. I couldn't believe it. In a matter of hours, we had gone from discussing something troubling to setting up an appointment with a breast surgeon.

"Of course, you can absolutely have your pick of doctors, but I cannot recommend this team enough," she said. "You would be in excellent hands."

I didn't know how to respond because I wasn't quite ready to receive this information. I was still in absolute shock and teetering on, *There is* no way *this is happening. There's no chance this is real. It can't be.* ·

I looked over at John and saw the shock on his face. He is always a calm and steady presence. He is truly unflappable. I think I've seen him *really* cry maybe three times. But I had never seen him like he was that day. He's always been so methodical, even-handed, and centered. He's always my rock. And for once, we were self-destructing together.

While John was a silent crier, I was still loudly sobbing. "What do they expect to see with the biopsy?" I asked my doctor in a panic. "What are they looking for?"

What I didn't realize yet was that this biopsy wasn't actually meant to tell me whether or not I had cancer. Everyone already believed that would be the diagnosis, even if it hadn't been formally confirmed to me. Instead, they were looking for the pathology to inform them of the *type* of breast cancer, whether it was hormone positive, and whether it had spread to my lymph nodes.

As we got out of the car and walked back into the medical building, I thought: *What if we just leave? What if we just get in the car and drive home? What if we leave town in ignorant bliss, and deal with everything when we get back?*

Of course, it was a stupid thought, but I had a fleeting fantasy of wanting to go back to that morning when I didn't know what I knew now. If a breast cancer diagnosis fell in a forest and no one was there to hear it, did it really happen? I wasn't sure I was ready for everything to be real. I was too busy praying that I would get to have one more good day, good week, good vacation. I was so desperate to go back to my life where all of the wonderful things had been happening, where I was able to live without knowing this part of my future.

But that wasn't possible.

We went back in the building, and I changed into the familiar robe. No one was in the biopsy room yet, so I sat down in one of the chairs and continued to sob. I figured I had a few minutes, so I frantically called my friend Lauren B. She had been through breast cancer a year prior, so I turned to her immediately for a shoulder to cry on. Lauren's case involved surgery, chemo, and radiation, so I figured she would be able to give me the most valuable insight as I was trying to process the road ahead of me. This is not the same Lauren as Lauren R., who I called from the Houston airport. I have so many friends named Lauren who have had breast cancer that I need to distinguish them with initials.

I pulled up her contact with hands shaking. When she answered, I rushed into an explanation of what had transpired throughout the day. I rambled on that I was pretty sure I had breast cancer, and that the doctors seemed pretty sure too. I started rattling off chaotic and panicked questions. But I couldn't make sense of the words coming out of my mouth, let alone her answers.

"Just try to remain calm. We're going to talk it through, and you can ask me anything you want. But for right now, let's get you through the biopsy," Lauren B. said.

"It's very loud," she warned me. "Like a nail gun. And just know that before they start, they are going to give you numbing medication. They're going to inject it, which doesn't feel great, but you're going to want it."

Having a needle—even before the actual biopsy instruments—inserted into my breast was not something I was looking forward to. But it beat the alternative, which was not having any numbing medication.

"Ask the nurses if they have any Ativan or anything to help you calm down in the meantime." We hung up, after I promised to call her back as soon as it was over. I felt a twinge of comfort as I sat there. Not because I had received any good news (far from it), but because I had someone who knew exactly what I was feeling in that moment. For the first time all day, I didn't feel alone in my swirl of emotions.

At that point, two women walked into the room and started explaining how the biopsy was going to work. They asked me to lie down on the table with my right arm over my head. As they were positioning me, I turned to the radiologist, who had also entered the room, and asked, "Is it possible it could be something else?"

She paused and looked at the other women before replying, "Honey. It's cancer."

That was it. The words I knew to be true but hadn't yet heard. The comforting feeling vanished, and an onslaught of pure terror came washing over me. I started sobbing yet again, but this time it was guttural. I was starting to grieve right there on that table.

As they began preparing me for the numbing medication, I stared up at the ceiling while tears continued to stream down my face. I realized I had been crying for hours into the same disposable mask we were still required to wear in hospitals. A sopping wet mask felt like a bit of insult to injury.

I looked around thinking, *Isn't everyone else in here going to freak out too? I just found out in this room that I have cancer!* But then I remembered that this was the breast center. Everyone in here probably had to deal with breast cancer patients every single day. To them this was normal.

There was some more conversation, looking over the imagery, and then it was time to get started. Well, Lauren B. was right. It is not fun to have a needle inserted into your breast. In addition to the unpleasant needle, the lidocaine itself burns. I thought, *This already sucks and they haven't even started.* Because this was a triple biopsy, I needed quite a bit of numbing. I flinched and sucked in my breath with each stick.

Lauren B. was right about the biopsy too. It is unnervingly loud. Both loud and uncomfortable. I would certainly say that combined with the emotional weight I was carrying, it was one of the worst moments of my life. I remember every painstaking second of that experience.

While it was happening I thought, *I did not sign up for this today.* I had assumed I was just coming in for a mammogram. I had mentally prepared myself to receive bad news (although it turned out I was woefully unprepared), but I hadn't anticipated that this was what it would be like, a fast-moving train of tests, doctors, reports, and follow-up appointments in which there wasn't a minute to spare. I'd had no idea at the start of that day that this was going to become such a harrowing experience.

In reality, I was lucky that I was able to get it all done in the same day. According to the American Cancer Society, about 8 to 10 percent of women are sent for a biopsy after their mammogram. Sometimes they have to wait days for it to be scheduled, then wait more days for the results.

The procedure felt like it was taking forever. But in reality, I have absolutely no idea how long I was on that table. An hour? Two hours? Forty-five minutes? What I was very well aware of, however, was being in an uncomfortable position for a long time. My arm was falling asleep, my nose was itching, and I was still in a damp mask. I wanted to scream and jump out of my skin. I couldn't take this much longer. I needed to get out of that room and see my husband again. We needed to start wrapping our heads around my foreseeable future.

When I was finally done, I put the dreaded robe back on. I wasn't allowed to get dressed or leave just yet, and I didn't understand why. It was probably explained to me, but I was barely able to hear information, let alone process it. I shuffled from room to room without seeing or hearing anything around me. I finally found my way back to the breast center waiting room (not the lobby, where John was).

It was the very end of the day—dinnertime. The lights in the building were half-off, and I sat there alone, watching the nurses and doctors leave for the day. I started my guttural sobs again. One of the passing nurses said, "Is everything all right, sweetheart?" and I said the words out loud for the first time: "No! I just found out I have breast cancer!"

One Thing

You might hear a lot about the four breast cancer stages.
Here's what they're talking about.

How will my doctor decide my stage?				
Stage	1	2	3	4
Tumor size	Less than 2 cm	2–5 cm	5 cm and larger	Any size
Lymph node	Not affected	Few armpit nodes may be affected.	More than 10 nodes may be affected.	Any number of nodes may be affected.
Cancer spread	Confined to breast area, not outside	Confined to breast area, not outside	Confined to breast area, not outside	Spread to any other part of the body

Sources:

breastcancerhub.org/breast-cancer/types-breast-cancer

dcodecare.com/about-cancer/breast-cancer/overview

One More Thing

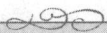

Not all appointments go the way you hope they will. If you can enlist a friend or a loved one to wait with you, it might make all the difference. If you don't have someone to come with you in person, have someone standing by on the phone.

This can feel like a big ask, but I've found that people are more than happy to jump in and help however they can. These requests often go best if you're very specific about what you need and what the possibilities are. Here's a sample script:

> Hi! I've got a big appointment coming up on Tuesday that I'm nervous about. Do you think you'd have time to go with me? The appointment is at eleven a.m. downtown and it will probably take about an hour, a lot of which will be time sitting around waiting. I'd love it if you'd come along to hold my hand and read magazines with me. If it goes well, I'll take us out to lunch after! And if it doesn't go well, I'd be grateful if you'd give me a hug and take me home.

Or:

> Hey! Would you be able to block out twelve to one p.m. on Tuesday to be around if I need to talk? I might be getting big news at my appointment and I'd love to know if you're around and up for celebrating with me, or letting me cry!

If enlisting a friend isn't an option, there are helplines you can call for support in many forms, whether you're looking for financial aid or a patient navigator (a person who helps patients navigate the health care system and access the services and care they need). One is the Susan G. Komen Breast Care Helpline, which you can reach either by phone at 877-465-6636 or by email at helpline@komen.org.

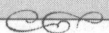

CHAPTER FIVE

Who Do I Tell?

I felt like I was slipping into a black hole where I couldn't see in any direction. I called my friend Lauren B. back from the little waiting room. "It's cancer," I said. "It is breast cancer. They're sure of it. I don't have the results back yet, but they're sure of it. I'm sure of it."

I was trying to let it sink in by saying the words out loud. Maybe if I said it enough times I would start to believe it. This was not a nightmare I could wake up from—it was one I was going to have to live through. I needed to know everything . . . how awful was chemo, was it the same for everyone, was I going to be throwing up the whole time, what was recovery like from surgery . . . ? I had a million and one questions.

As the lights at the center kept flicking off around me, I thought, *Yep, that feels right.* It was a metaphor for how I was feeling, sitting in the robe, on the phone with Lauren B. It was as if everything inside me was shutting off along with the lights.

Lauren B. was very calm while she explained, "I had triple negative breast cancer—which in the world of breast cancer is not the one you want. Not that there is any kind you *do* want."

This might be a good time to remind everyone that I'm *not* a doctor, even though I prematurely glance at screens in the ultrasound room. But I soon learned that triple negative means that your cancer cells do not have estrogen or progesterone receptors, and they're also negative for HER2, or human epidermal growth factor receptor 2. Hence the term *triple negative*. One of the reasons why triple negative breast cancer (TNBC) is considered a less favorable diagnosis is because starving the tumor of those hormones isn't a possibility. And having fewer long-term treatment options often leads to a poorer prognosis.

On the other hand, if you're hormone positive, it means (again: I am not a doctor! Don't quote me!) that your cancer cells *do* have hormone receptors, and they grow from signals sent through estrogen, progesterone, or both. This actually makes long-term treatment viable because you can take medications and get infusions that shut down your hormone production. This doesn't mean it's not possible for cancer to return, but you have options to mitigate the risk.

I was trying to learn all this information in real time, and it was *a lot* to take in. As Lauren B. went on to explain chemo treatments, I tried to take mental notes.

"The worst is a treatment called the 'red devil,'" she said. "The red devil is hard. The name says it all."

Noted. I didn't want to be triple negative and the red devil sounded like a no thank-you. Lauren B. then added, "It truly is awful, but it will save your life. I don't know whether you will need chemo or not, but if you do, you'll probably receive that treatment."

Fine, maybe it wasn't a complete no thank-you to the red devil.

Maybe it was a necessary evil that I'd learn to live with. But I wasn't exactly looking forward to it.

"The only thing that I can definitely tell you is to please, *please* not google any of this," Lauren B. added. She advised me to talk to the doctors instead, to get the pathology back instead of jumping to conclusions, and to trust my team.

I understood this, even as I was shaking with impatience and fear, waiting to find out my results. If it was officially cancer, this would tell me the type of cancer I had and how bad it was. I tried to heed these words of advice, even though it was easier said than done. Of course I wanted to start googling things, but Google wasn't going to give me biopsy results, so I had to wait. I was going to have to keep waiting.

After I hung up with Lauren B., the tears kept coming. I wondered what the other women in the waiting room had heard. Was it just me who left with a cancer diagnosis? Or were there additional tears in the waiting room? I recalled the statistical likelihood that I wasn't the only woman at the center who would go home that day with bad news.

At this point I was given my little plastic bag of belongings and finally told I could change and leave for the night. Putting my clothes back on felt like an insurmountable task. I didn't know up from down and I had to put *jeans* on?

When I eventually changed and walked out to the lobby, I saw John still sitting there. It had been more than six hours since he'd first walked in with me. His eyes were red from tears. His face was the most somber I'd ever seen it. It was sinking in for both of us.

When this day had started, our focus was still on going to Paris and hopefully crossing off a major medical scare. We were hoping we could enjoy our trip with peace of mind and have a great time without worry. Walking back into that waiting room, it was clear our world had changed forever. The fear, the sadness, the hopelessness, the disbelief . . . the utter despair. It all came crashing over us every few minutes.

As we drove home, more tears spurted out of me as John and I asked ourselves: What do we do now? Where do we go from here? Are we going on our trip tomorrow? What is the plan? And who should we tell?

Everyone was going to find out soon enough, but who should I tell today? So far, the circle of people who knew was pretty small: John, Joanna, my parents, some close friends who were breast cancer survivors. Who would be next?

I ruled out discussing this with the kids yet. I needed to have a lot more information so that I could answer their questions and reassure them I was going to be okay. So far, I had not let myself consider a world where I was *not* going to be okay, and I wanted to be able to back that up with a full diagnosis. I started making a list of people I had to call; my brother was at the top because my parents already knew.

But before I could do that, I had to talk to my mother again. We just sat on the phone and cried for a long while before she said, "You're canceling your trip, right?"

"Definitely not—I am one hundred percent going. What else am I supposed to do while I wait for test results and future doctor appointments?"

My mother went silent, which was a clear sign of disapproval, but she ultimately said I needed to do what felt right. And leaving town instead of wallowing while playing the waiting game felt extremely right.

I had spoken to my doctor and she had encouraged me to go on vacation while the dust settled. She would contact me as soon as my biopsy results were in, and at the moment, there were no follow-up appointments booked yet. That was that—it was decided.

When John and I got home, it was hard to walk in the door, to ask our kids normal questions like how school went and if they needed help with homework. I mean, it was very, *very* hard. My mind was on another planet and my eyes were so red I could barely see straight. After they went to sleep, I started making phone calls.

It had been an insane twelve hours so far, but I knew I needed to spend the next few on the phone. Aside from John, Joanna, my parents, and a few close friends (Christina, Lauren R., Lauren B.), no one else knew that these appointments had even happened. I hadn't told anyone else that I'd discovered a lump, and certainly not that I had been to the breast center that day. This news was going to come as a shock to anyone I told. I knew the feeling; I hadn't been expecting it either.

When I called my brother, I could barely get the words out. He is *not* a dramatic person (I received all those genes), but I could hear the wind being knocked out of him. There are no other siblings, so the two of us have always had a special bond. Neither of us could handle a life-threatening situation involving the other.

The next few days were tough, and I had to make some difficult decisions. That was the course of action every day for the next couple of weeks, but the first few days were paramount. I had to figure out if I was going to tell someone or not, and then think about how they might react when they did find out. Would they be offended that I had been keeping it from them? Would they understand I needed to move slowly because it was hard saying the words out loud and reliving the emotion every single time?

I went back to planning mode and made a list of who I was going to call immediately, who I was going to tell after our trip, and who else I needed to make sure to contact directly before they saw it publicly or found out from someone else. I also knew I was going to need to arm myself with information, because I was surely going to get a lot of questions. Which was fair because I too had a lot of questions. I didn't know how big my tumors were, what stage of cancer I had, or what my course of treatment would look like. There were just so many unknowns.

But there was one question I needed an answer to right away.

For the third time that day, I called Dr. Kurtz. (I am extremely lucky to have a very responsive primary care doctor. I know that's not true of every physician's office, but I'd encourage anyone going through this to reach out to their doctor's office as much as they feel called to. The doctor won't pick up if they're in the middle of something else. And if it's taking a really long time to get answers even to important questions, it might be time to look for another doctor.)

I asked her nervously, "Do I have any reason to believe that this isn't treatable?"

"No, we do not have any reason to believe that," she replied.

I breathed a sigh of relief. (The bar for my relief was now pretty low. I had just been told I had cancer, but at least I was going to be able to treat it.) With that knowledge, I could at least let people know that bare minimum of information: *We have no reason to believe this isn't treatable.* I tried to steel myself with those words even as I repeated them out loud. I reminded myself over and over that the survival rate for breast cancer is very high, and I was *going to be* on the surviving side. I would go through any treatment necessary, and I was going to live a long cancer-free life.

Was I scared as hell? Yes.

Was I anxious to know what the rest of the year—and the rest of my life—would look like? Yes, of course.

I was going to have to sift through and process a lot of fears and unknowns, but death was simply not going to be one of them.

I tried to end my terrible day with a little bit of resolve: I was absolutely, positively going to beat cancer. I was determined. And while there was nothing I could immediately do to put this plan in motion, it felt huge. This was going to be my North Star every single day because I knew that if I started to let the fear creep in, I probably wasn't going to be successful at keeping the actual cancer at bay.

So, I ended the day pumping myself up with a pep talk: *I can do this, I'm going to do this, I'm not afraid to do this.*

But even after my mental pep talk, I woke up the next morning wanting to believe that it was just a bad dream. Try as I might, my first thoughts were, *I have cancer. I am a person living with cancer. I am a cancer patient now.*

One Thing

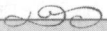

Deciding who to tell about your diagnosis, and when, is a deeply personal choice. You don't owe anyone an immediate explanation, and you should take your time to process your own feelings and thoughts. But above all, do not feel guilty if you do *not* want to tell people. You might want to share your news with everyone or with some people, or you might want to tell no one at all. I'm a list maker, so I wrote down the groups of people I wanted to tell. Do whatever feels right to you.

I identified the core people in my life who needed to know first based on either family or friend relationships, people who had to know for practical reasons like our nanny and work colleagues, and people who I felt I could identify with and lean on for support.

Hoda Kotb was one of the first people I told that I had cancer. We were organizing her office for the *Today* show. I pulled her aside and I told her. She gave me the biggest hug and some advice: "You have been moving too fast, and the universe is telling you to slow down, and sometimes you have to listen to what the universe is saying."

Then she said, "I beat it and you're going to beat it too. You're going to be one of the survivors along with us."

Hoda was such a source of support for me throughout the entire process. Witnessing a cancer survivor thriving, looking amazing, feeling amazing, and doing all the things brought me a lot of hope. She was a huge, huge inspiration to me and a source of great comfort. Try to identify who in your orbit is most like Hoda, and tell that person.

You will not be able to share the news with everyone in person—I even had to tell my mother over the phone. But regardless of how they happen, initial conversations can be at your own pace, on your own terms. There is no golden rule or guidebook for how to handle this huge moment in your life. Once you have opened your diagnosis up to a few, the next handful of people will start to come into focus, and then the next. I even recall moving to text for certain friends because I just didn't have the bandwidth for another phone conversation. Once I felt confident I had told the majority of people in my life, I went ahead and posted the news on so- cial media. That's not something everyone decides to do, but for me, it was a critical part of sharing my story, and one that has changed the course of my life.

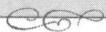

CHAPTER SIX

The Diagnosis

John, the kids, and I were set to fly to California right after my unofficial diagnosis. It was the start of spring break, and we were taking Stella (who was eleven) and Sutton (who was eight) to visit John's mom in Laguna Beach for the week. John and I were then set to fly to Paris for our own vacation. In my constant calculation about who to tell, I decided not to share the news with my mother-in-law yet because I didn't want to burden her with this information while she was taking care of the kids. Dropping a bombshell like that didn't seem fair, especially because the kids didn't know yet either.

As I rode in the car with my family on the way to the Nashville International Airport, I was worried my thoughts would betray me. I looked around the car anxiously, feeling like I was living a lie. Stella and Sutton were happily chatting about going to the beach and everything they wanted to do in California, and here I was holding this huge secret that was going to impact their lives in an enormous way.

I texted Lauren B. from the back seat, because even after all our conversations the night before, I didn't know how to push through that moment.

"I'm in the car with the kids heading to the airport right now," I told her. "We're headed to California to drop them off and then we're going to Europe."

"That's good," she said. "It will be a nice distraction, and you won't be able to travel for a long time once the treatments start."

My anxiety spiked through the roof. "What do you mean? Why?" I asked.

"Well, during chemo, you're not really going to be able to travel because of the risk of infection. And then if you do radiation, that's going to be every day. It's going to make it pretty difficult to travel, at least for a while."

I'd been receiving a lot of rapid-fire information, but this was the first major realization of how life as I knew it was going to dramatically change. This was the first moment that I thought my quality of life was going to change dramatically. I traveled *all the time*. I couldn't fathom going into another lockdown where I wasn't able to go anywhere. We were coming out of COVID and things could finally happen again. I didn't want to go back into a prison, where this time I was the only one in jail. It was just another crushing reality, another thing that I wouldn't have thought about a day prior. Another thing cancer was going to take from me that I hadn't seen coming.

I was already terrified of how chemo would make me feel (and look), and now I had to add these life restrictions to the list. Admittedly, all my chemo knowledge came from TV and movies. Which looked like it involved sitting in uncomfortable chairs, in a big room, attached to an IV for hours. And everyone was *always* throwing up. But none of these shows ever mentioned not being able to go anywhere or be around people. Of course, I had assumed my immunity would be compromised, but I never connected that with being on house arrest.

By the time we arrived at the airport, I had figured out that what scared me most about cancer wasn't the prospect of dying. It was losing my life in a different way. It was the quality of my life plummeting that started to scare me the most. I was thinking, *Am I just going to be sick all the time? Am I going to be confined to my bed? Or worse, a hospital bed?* There was no crystal ball for this, so these questions swirled in my mind without answers. That was my first dose of realizing that in the weeks and months to come, I wasn't just going to be battling an illness—I was going to be battling plenty of mental demons too.

This fear dripped in my veins as we checked in at the airport ticket desk and passed through security. When we entered the lounge, I noticed those private phone-booth-like areas where you can work or take a phone call. I signaled to John that I was heading over there, and I dipped into one so I could call Lauren B. instead of texting her a thousand more questions.

"Tell me exactly what you mean," I said, "that I can't go anywhere, that I can't travel. Does that mean *anywhere*? Can I be on an airplane? What if I drove? How far could I go in a car?" I was trying to ask her everything.

Lauren B. sighed. "I know it's a lot to take in. Honestly, you're going to just take it a day at a time and talk to your doctors about what you can and cannot do."

"If I can't go anywhere, I will go crazy," I told her. "I won't just be a cancer patient. I will also become a mental patient. If I can't do anything, I will be out of my head."

Thank goodness I was in a soundproof booth because I couldn't stop crying. I looked over at my kids sitting around the corner from me, and I thought again about how I was harboring this huge secret from them. They were so blissfully ignorant. I couldn't destroy that ignorance yet. I wanted them to stay carefree and happy for as long as possible. This was just going to be my problem for now.

On the flight to California, I kept thinking about how I was currently in the small window of time before everything would begin. The rush of treatment options and surgery dates wouldn't start until I was back in Nashville. This was the time when everything was suspended in midair. Was I going to obsess over what was to come, or would I be able to live in the moment and have a good time? I imagined the latter would be impossible, but I could find pockets between my obsessive thoughts. If the plane ride was any indication, I would have moments when I felt briefly okay, and then low, crushing moments when I silently sobbed again.

There is no data to support that cancer hurts. The opposite is in fact true. Cancer doesn't hurt and can be imperceptible until it's too late. But I couldn't stop myself from thinking I felt it deeply. Yes, there were the tumors I could feel, but there was something else. As soon as I knew I had cancer growing inside my body, I couldn't stop myself from feeling it at all times.

After we arrived in California, John and I stayed with his mom for a couple of days to make sure that the kids were acclimated before we left town. I was constantly on the phone during that period talking to Joanna and the few friends who knew: Leah,

Christina, Merritt, Marla, Stevie, and all the Laurens. Because my mother-in-law didn't know about anything, I said I had work calls and took walks around the block. Finally, two days later, I got the call I was waiting for.

Dr. Kurtz had the results of my biopsy. She had rushed the tests so that we could discuss them before I left the country. Before we got into the details, we were able to cross the big one off our list in black-and-white terms: Yes, I definitely had breast cancer. Invasive mammary carcinoma, to be exact. The five-year survival rate is almost 100 percent if you catch it early. If it's spread to other tissue in the area, that drops to 86 percent. And if it's spread to other parts of your body, it's 28 percent.

I was going to need to meet with my soon-to-be oncologist to review what each line item meant, but there were a few results that provided some key information. For starters, there were two sizable tumors, one measuring three centimeters and the other measuring just under two centimeters. I held my breath for the next piece of news . . . I was ER/PR positive. Meaning I wasn't triple negative. This was a relief, as I recalled my conversation with Lauren B. Being ER/PR positive would mean extra treatment, but at least I would be *able* to receive extra treatment. With breast cancer, there is always a risk of recurrence—you are constantly living in the shadow of that possibility. So the potential for any additional safeguard beyond primary treatment helps tremendously.

For the last bit of crucial information: The pathology came back that my lymph nodes were clear. That meant the cancer was localized in my right breast, and had not spread to my lymph nodes. That was the best news of all. My doctor advised that I talk about this with Dr. Park, who would be my oncologist. I hadn't yet met

Dr. Park, but Dr. Kurtz strongly recommended that he be in charge of my care. She said that Dr. Park would be reviewing these results to determine my course of treatment, advise on surgery options, and answer all my questions better than anyone else I could talk to.

I had already decided that I was going to opt for a double mastectomy no matter what the other options were. My anxiety was not going to let me entertain the notion of a lumpectomy even if that was a possibility, and I didn't see the point of a single mastectomy. If I could grow cancer in my right breast, I could probably grow it in my left breast—so I wanted *everything* removed just in case.

"I completely understand that logic," she replied when I explained this to her, "but talk to Dr. Park. Work through all of your options, and figure out what you want to do."

I was willing to take any good news at this point. I kept reminding myself of it. The cancer was not in my lymph nodes, and I was hormone positive. These were good things in a sea of bad things, and I hung on to that information like a life preserver in the ocean.

One Thing

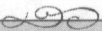

Please listen to Lauren B.'s advice:

Do not google.

Talk to your doctors. Talk to people who are undergoing treatment for cancer. Talk to cancer survivors. Read books by survivors, doctors, and experts. Join online support groups. But do not google.

Get information, advice, and encouragement from survivors, experts, and books. But googling will lead you down a dark path full of anxiety and sleepless nights. With all due respect to Google, of course.

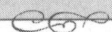

CHAPTER SEVEN

Paris

I was more stressed than usual saying goodbye to the kids, but John and I managed to pack up and head off to LAX. We would soon be on our way to Paris—I just wished I could have felt more excited.

Once we arrived at the airport and got settled, I found a quiet corner of the lounge to make a few phone calls. Before I got on the plane I needed to tell some very important people what was going on: the new owners of The Home Edit, Hello Sunshine.

My very first call was to Hello Sunshine's CEO, Sarah Harden. I couldn't believe that a couple of weeks prior we were opening bottles of champagne to celebrate our acquisition, and now I needed to tell her this horrible news. My second call was to Reese Witherspoon, the founder of Hello Sunshine. These two women had not just supported The Home Edit for all these years, but they'd supported me personally. I simply could *not* let them down.

My calls continued as I walked toward my gate on the moving sidewalk. Maureen Polo, the head of direct-to-consumer at Hello Sunshine (where The Home Edit sat in the organization), was my third call. Because Maureen specifically managed our business, I think I was most nervous to tell her about my diagnosis. But after speaking with these remarkable women, all my nerves melted away. They were each so fiercely supportive, and adamant that my health needed to come first. I still couldn't help but apologize for the disruption and promise I would still be able to function as usual (such a stereotypically feminine thing to do . . . men would never), but they put each of my protests to rest.

I realized that day that I was sharing my diagnosis with more and more people. With each new person I told, I was further putting it into the universe that I had cancer. Admitting it to myself was one thing. Admitting it out loud to individual people was totally different. Passing on the information almost made it feel like the problem was growing. It was no longer something that I could just whisper to myself. It was becoming a known entity. It was becoming legitimate. This was quickly becoming not just my secret.

The first few days of our trip were exceptionally hard. The shock had worn off, and now I was just left with a grim understanding of the battle ahead of me. John and I took long walks around Paris, as though getting twenty-five thousand steps was going to shrink my disease. I wasn't much of a conversationalist on those walks. I was either silent or speculating about what the near future would be like. I couldn't get out of my very depressed state. I was starting to mourn the life I'd known just a few days ago. We would do normal things like go shopping, and I would say to John, "Why even buy this? Where am I going in it? Am I ever leaving the house again?"

At that time, everything felt so bleak and so dreary that it was hard to escape the feeling of doom.

Our good friends Matt and Lauren R. decided to make a last-minute trip to see us in Paris because they live not too far away, in Switzerland.

"We're going to be there," Lauren told me.

I cried tears of gratitude imagining being around Lauren, who knew what this moment was like for me, and Matt, who knew what this moment was like for John.

We were on our way to meet them for breakfast, and I had a genuine pep in my step for the first time all week. Standing at a busy intersection on Boulevard Saint-Germain, I spotted Lauren waiting for us on the other side of the street. The second the light turned green I took off running to hug her. And then I ran into the café to hug Matt too (I presume John was chasing me down to make sure I didn't get hit in the traffic). Seeing them and being with them changed my mood entirely. That was the turning point in our trip.

Having Matt and Lauren R. there made things feel slightly normal again. It felt so good just to be able to *laugh*. I hadn't laughed since I was diagnosed, and I was kind of worried I wasn't going to be able to laugh again until this was behind me. So getting a few brief moments when I was able to forget that I had cancer, even for a second, felt so good. There were even a couple of meals when I could block out the dread inside me and have a regular conversation.

It was during the latter half of my time in Paris, after seeing Matt and Lauren R., that I started to feel stronger and less afraid. I began to realize how many women in my life had been through breast cancer, and how much they had thrived despite it. These women had kicked cancer's butt.

For the first time, I thought, *Fuck this. I am going crush cancer too.*

Our hotel room had a vintage typewriter in it that I'm pretty sure was just meant to be decorative, but there was paper, so I loaded it in and put the typewriter to the test. I didn't realize that my anger was going to come out through my fingers so forcefully, but I started slamming down the keys, writing: *I'm not afraid of cancer.* Then I wrote it again. Then I added, *Cancer should be afraid of me.*

I wanted to make sure I believed it. I needed to believe that I wasn't afraid of cancer, and sometimes truly believing takes writing something down or saying it out loud—putting it out into the world in order for it to resonate. I didn't know it then, but that was my metamorphosis.

For days, I had been plagued with asking, "Why me?" But in that moment, I thought: *Why not me? I can do this. I will do this. I have all the resources and help in the world: the best medical care; the most supportive husband; the greatest family, friends, and coworkers. If one in eight women gets cancer, maybe better for it to be me than someone else with fewer resources.* I had the will, I had the fortitude, and I had a platform where I could try to make a difference. I suddenly felt empowered. *I will beat this disease, and I will make my cancer purposeful. I'm going to talk about it openly, I'm going to share my experience from start to finish, and if I can help save just one person's life, it will have been worth it.*

I made a commitment then and there to not battle privately. I wanted to share my story with as many people as possible in the hope that it would reach whoever needed it. Maybe it would encourage women to get their annual mammogram, or speak up if they found something on their own like I had. Maybe it would resonate with people who were experiencing the same thing. And maybe—hopefully—if people could see that I was crushing cancer, it would help inspire the same confidence in themselves. Just like my friends had inspired me.

I wasn't going to waste time being sick. I was going to document every moment—both good and bad. This was about a lot more than me, and I was going to make sure of it.

The last couple of days of our trip I had renewed energy. Like someone had given me marching orders and said, "Go." I was going to head home, meet with my oncologist, and make a plan. Cancer was going to be no match for me.

One Thing

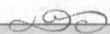

When it came time to share the news of my diagnosis with people at work, I was pretty anxious about how to initiate the conversation, how much information I should include, and even the order in which I should make the phone calls. My friends who had been through this previously all varied dramatically in terms of how they handled each situation, and I couldn't find much guidance online, so if this is at all helpful, here is how I approached the news with my company.

As I mentioned, the first three conversations I needed to have outside of immediate friends and family were with Sarah Harden, Maureen Polo, and Reese Witherspoon.

I decided not to beat around the bush at all. As soon as they answered, I dove right into why I was calling them. "I wanted you to be among the first people I've shared this news with. I have breast cancer," I said. In almost all instances there was a sharp intake of breath on the other end of the line. It was then when I jumped in with a few critical details I wanted to convey immediately:

1. My case is treatable and will begin with surgery as soon as possible. Further treatment will depend on a host of variables.

2. I am not going anywhere.

3. You will be the first to know as I have more information.

After I had spoken to everyone in leadership at Hello Sunshine and The Home Edit, I considered how I would disseminate the news to the company at large. I really wanted everyone to hear it from me rather than someone else. We had a company-wide meeting coming up, so I (rather shakily) stood in front of everyone to tell them about the news with the key details anchoring my speech. It was critical to me that everyone could look into my eyes and see nothing but strength and resolve. It mattered to me, and I think it mattered to them too.

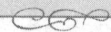

CHAPTER EIGHT

And So It Begins

When we landed back in Los Angeles, John picked up the kids to head home to Nashville while I stayed a few extra days for work. These additional days meant I would not go back immediately for doctor appointments (for which I was grateful), but I knew this trip would be coming to an end shortly. Because I was there for a brand campaign shoot, I needed to temporarily shake off the stress and reality of the past week, and somehow put on my game face. I was thinking, *I have to refocus my energy and get back into work mode*. To be honest, I love work mode—it's where I thrive. But I was finding it hard to dive back in without all the unknowns rattling around in my head: *Is this the last work trip I'm going to go on for a long time? Is this the last trip, period? Will I be able to work at all anymore?*

I *had* to push those thoughts out of my mind, which involved some of the hardest mental gymnastics I've ever done. My doctor would be able to give me some of the answers once I got home, so truly, there was no benefit to letting my questions enter the spin cycle of my brain. Every now and then, in moments like these, it was nice to be able to take back some of the power from this illness. To decide it was worthy of no airtime. I couldn't foresee the future, but I could promise myself that on this particular day, I was done spiraling.

The days spent in L.A. were bittersweet. I wanted to hang on to every last minute before reality crept in. But I also knew that I had to get back to Nashville and get this show on the road. Time away meant time wasted, and because my health was a ticking time bomb, I figured I should probably head back and start to defuse it. I felt (as) ready (as I'd ever be).

Back in Nashville, I went right back into planning mode. It was finally time to take aggressive action; I wanted this cancer out of my body for good.

First things first: I met with my new oncologist, Dr. Park. He doesn't like it when patients call him Dr. Park; he prefers to be called Ben. He's the director of the Vanderbilt-Ingram Cancer Center and a doctor, like, twelve times over. Personally, I would make my children call me Dr. Shearer if I had been in medical school that long. But okay . . . I will sometimes (like, one out of ten times) call him Ben, but I just can't call a doctor saving my life by his first name.

John and I sat in Dr. Park's office in mid-March to thoroughly discuss the pathology that had come back from my biopsy. He first confirmed what Dr. Kurtz had already told me: I was hormone positive and HER2 negative. But there was a lot of additional, very specific information that my biopsied tumor provided. I learned that my cancer was aggressive and fast-moving; I had high histological grade 3 tumors. And based on my Oncotype score (essentially, how likely your cancer is to return), I had a high risk of reoccurrence. This meant that I would likely benefit from chemotherapy and ongoing hormone therapy. But because my lymph nodes were clean, and the cancer seemed localized in my right breast, it potentially meant that *maybe* treatment would be minimal. But no matter what came next, the first step in this process was going to be surgery.

"I want a double mastectomy," I said. "I want everything gone. If I can get cancer on my right side, then I can get cancer on my left side."

A lot of people ask why I opted for a double mastectomy as opposed to a different surgery, so I want to make it clear to everyone reading. My doctors did not tell me I *needed* a double mastectomy. A single mastectomy would have been an option, because the tumors were only on my right side. It was my choice to remove both of my breasts. It's a very personal decision that you make alongside your doctor, but this was what I wanted. The most important calculation in this journey is, of course, what your doctor advises, but beyond that, listen to your head, your gut, your heart.

Then Dr. Park asked me, "What are you most afraid of?"

That was an interesting question because it wasn't death. "Chemo," I said. "I'm most afraid of chemo."

"There's a *chance* that you won't need chemotherapy, or at least you'd only do minimal chemotherapy," Dr. Park said after I told him that was keeping me up at night. "We have to get through the surgery first, remove the tumors, and assess the situation," he continued. "It might just be a few rounds of abbreviated chemotherapy, but we'll know more soon. We won't know about radiation until then as well."

"That would be the best news I've heard since March eighth," I said.

"You will, however, definitely need endocrine therapy in the future," he confirmed.

The next thing he told me, I held on to for dear life: "I believe that your cancer is not just treatable, but curable."

Curable.

Please, please let it be so.

Next, I met with my breast surgeon, Dr. Meszoely, and my plastic surgeon, Dr. Perdikis, so we could schedule a surgery date and determine my options for reconstruction. The plan was that I was going to go direct to implant following my double mastectomy, which meant it was all going to be one procedure. So far, this felt like the best-case scenario amid many much worse scenarios. Maybe this process would be swifter than I had imagined. Maybe this would be behind me before I knew it.

My surgery was scheduled for April 8. We were moving fast, which I appreciated. I've always been someone who acts immediately. If I have my marching orders, I want it done yesterday so I can cross it off my list. I started making preparations in the lead-up to my surgery date. My mother was planning to fly in and stay with me throughout recovery; my dad would follow a week or so after. John would be with me at the hospital with our friend Krista, and Joanna would be on standby.

But the most important puzzle piece still needed to be addressed. I hadn't told my children. I wanted to save them from this information until the last possible moment because I didn't want them to carry fear any longer than necessary. There was no reason to inflict on them the sense of dread that John and I were feeling. I wanted them to know I was going into surgery, but that I would be out the next day with nothing to worry about.

I waited until the night before. Sitting them down, I said, "I have to tell you something, but I want you to know that this is not something I'm afraid of." Then I said, "I have breast cancer." The shocked silence filled the air for a moment before Stella broke down, and Sutton got tearful. I was quick to explain that I was having surgery the next day to get the cancer removed and completely out of my body.

I was careful with the words I used because I didn't want to promise outcomes I couldn't guarantee, nor did I want to alarm them with information that didn't offer the full picture. I leaned on what I knew was true: I was not afraid of surgery, I did not have the type of cancer that we had to be really scared about, and I felt certain the surgery would work. We didn't need to be afraid, we just needed to handle the situation.

I tried to relate my surgery to that of our beloved dog, Emmett, who had to have some cancerous growths removed from his body. Emmett had a lump. Mommy had a lump. We both needed surgeries. Was that a very simplified description? Yes. But I needed it for myself as much as for the kids. My prognosis was far too big and overwhelming to process otherwise. Stella and Sutton were pretty rocked by the news. I would never suggest the best way to talk to your kids, but I would recommend talking to them when they have the space to experience a range of emotions without feeling self-conscious. For me, this meant telling them at home, when no guests were around, and doing so after school, when I knew we'd have plenty of time to talk and wouldn't feel rushed. It wasn't easy. Even though telling them was painful, I emphasized that I was going to be fine and that it was 100 percent going to be okay. Something I believed deep in my core.

I had never had surgery before, so for this major operation, an actual amputation, to be my first meant really diving in head-on. I was naturally nervous, but there was a calm about me that I can't quite explain. I had already accepted this and actually felt ready to have this surgery in my rearview mirror.

After we checked in at the hospital, John and I sat in the waiting room with a lot of nervous energy. My mother had given me a small silver four-leaf clover that I clutched in the palm of my hand. Pretty soon they called me back to prep me for surgery. I didn't want to leave John in the waiting room because the last time I had done that, our lives had turned upside down. But they assured us that he could come back before my surgery started. He would also be notified every step along the way, and alerted when I was in the recovery room.

I walked tentatively into the room they assigned me and saw a blue gown, a blue cap, and yellow socks. This was getting very real. I quickly undressed and got onto the bed wearing my hospital gown. The nurse entered the room as soon as I'd sat down and said she would be taking care of me. I had the usual check of vitals, and then the dreaded IV that went right into the hand. I swear, that is the worst part of surgery. The next couple of hours were a blur of nurses and doctors coming in and out, introducing themselves, and asking me the same three questions: (1) Can you tell me your name? (2) Date of birth? (3) And in your own words, what procedure are you getting today?

"I'm having a bilateral mastectomy with reconstruction."

After I answered each set of questions, they would sign their name on my right breast with a black Sharpie. I couldn't help but laugh every time they did that. Has medical science not progressed beyond a Sharpie signature on the skin?

Both of my surgeons, Dr. Perdikis and Dr. Meszoely, arrived and asked if I was ready to get started. I could answer honestly that I was. The anesthesiologist (the hero of any surgery tale) entered the room and gave me a rundown of what was expected. Of all the doctors he was the one I grilled: "Will I feel anything? How do I know it's working? Will you be able to tell if it's not working?"

As I was being wheeled to the operating room, I continued to pepper him with questions and only stopped short of a pinkie swear. He assured me I would feel nothing, and that if I did, he wasn't doing his job. Fair enough. The last thing I remember is that he said I would be unconscious for about four hours. Then it faded to black.

Turned out I was unconscious for double that.

One Thing

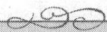

One of the common questions I get is how to decide between doctors when assembling a team. In my case, Dr. Kurtz recommended the team of doctors who cared for me, and I was *so* grateful to have her consult for me because I trust her implicitly. Not everyone has a primary care doctor to lead them in the right direction, so I tend to ask a few prodding questions when people want my advice.

1. Is there a particular doctor with whom you connected? A personal connection matters *a lot* when selecting a doctor. You need to be able to trust their advice and expertise, feel comfortable enough to speak up and ask questions, and have someone who can put you at ease during very difficult conversations.

2. Do any of the doctors in question have direct expertise connected to your specific cancer diagnosis?

3. Do you know any current or former patients you can ask?

4. Is there a hospital or office location that will make your life significantly easier? You're signing up for long-term care, treatments, and surgeries, and you will be visiting often. Don't make this experience any more stressful than it already is.

Once your team is in place, those early days of doctor appointments can be *very* overwhelming. You're meeting with so many people and receiving so much information. Try to write down all your questions so that you don't forget to get something answered. It also helps to have someone else in the room to take notes and capture the responses. It's very normal to be in a state of shock and not able to remember any given conversation. Deputize a partner, family member, or friend who can be in the room with you to document everything and make sure all your questions are answered.

This particular chapter has dealt with a lot of bumps (boulders?) in the road. In my case, I always leaned on the mantra "Trust your doctors and trust your gut." They work hand in hand. You might encounter forks in the road that seem scary, but your doctor and your gut will see you through. I had never needed much medical care beyond a flu shot, so this was very new to me. But accepting my new territory and allowing space for my naivete helped a lot. I didn't feel lost. . . . I just felt new. I was a willing participant in this journey, as I had already accepted my fate, but I need to be coached along—and to cross-check how I was feeling inside with the advice I was getting from experts.

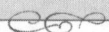

CHAPTER NINE

Complications

More than nine hours later, I woke up in the recovery room *very* out of it. John was sitting next to me trying to tell me something, and I'm pretty sure my doctor had visited me as well, but I couldn't say for sure. Why did I feel like there was something wrong? Was John telling me something was wrong? He kept asking me if I understood, but I had no idea what he was talking about.

My surgeon had indeed come in to speak to me already, but John had to re-explain the information, and then repeat it several times so that it sank in.

"They found cancer in your lymph nodes. It wasn't localized to your right breast; it spread," John said.

I didn't immediately understand what he was saying or what it meant. I was just trying to process the word *spread*. Even in my hazy state, I knew that was not a word you wanted to go along with cancer.

John continued, "You also weren't able to get your implants put in because your treatment plan will be different than expected. . . .

Dr. Perdikis will explain all this, but they had to put in breast expanders instead."

"Will I need chemo?" I asked.

"It sounds like yes . . . and radiation too," John said quietly. "And Dr. Perdikis said reconstruction would have to wait a year following radiation until you're healed from treatment."

This felt like diagnosis day all over again. I went into surgery thinking I had stage 1 breast cancer with tumors localized to my right breast. I woke up finding out that I was stage 2, with cancer that had spread through my lymphatic system. I knew that I had aggressive and fast-moving cancer, and I knew that I had a high risk of reoccurrence. So, this was definitely, most certainly going to make things much worse.

I was also staring down the barrel of lengthy treatment that I hadn't planned for. I would need to speak to Dr. Park about what that specifically involved, but I didn't anticipate a bunch of good news. My resolve, which I had worked so hard to cement, melted at that moment. It wasn't what I expected, of course. It wasn't in my plan. This was the first time I had to accept that when it comes to cancer, things can turn on a dime. This isn't a predictable disease. You can't be attached to a specific outcome because the path may very well lead you elsewhere. There also isn't time to question that path because you need to move forward quickly and decisively. Without a fully formulated plan, you just have to have faith that the path you're on is in fact the correct one. This is not exactly great if you're a type A control freak, but I was going to need to learn how to adapt.

Medicated as I was, for hours I had trouble absorbing all the new information. I thought, *I need to put this on the top shelf for a moment because I have to heal from surgery first.* Maybe it's the organizer in me, but I literally visualized putting this information into a labeled bin and placing it on the top shelf of my closet. It's the only way I knew how to compartmentalize the upcoming treatment, when I knew I had to first focus on recovering from a major operation. I needed to focus on healing and gaining my strength back, so I could fight like hell afterward. Because it certainly sounded like I was going to need to do just that.

There was a lot to process as doctors continued to come in and out of my hospital room. I didn't recognize any of them, not a single one. At one point I asked someone, "Did all of you operate on me? Why are there so many? So many . . ." as I drifted in and out of sleep.

When you come out of nine hours of anesthesia, you still feel pretty drugged. Nine-plus hours is a long time to be under. I just want to add a cautionary word here: *Do not use your phone after anesthesia.* My phone should have been taken away from me, locked up. John should have told me my phone was off to run errands because I would have believed him. I would have nodded and gone back to sleep. To everyone I sent a text to that day—April 8—I'm sure I need to apologize. There were missing letters, words, and punctuation, and a lot of unnecessary spaces. They were embarrassing to read back. Heed my warning.

I kept picking up my phone to reply to texts, and I was not quite able to keep it from slipping out of my hand. I had an 86 percent chance of living five more years, and a 60 percent chance of dropping my phone on my face. One doctor (I still had zero face recognition) tried talking to me and saw that I was half typing and half falling asleep, so he just backed slowly out of the room.

I also believed that there had been a curious emoji update in which every single icon had changed to a tiger's face—a tiger with heart eyes, a tiger laughing, a tiger surfing . . .

The next day, when I was feeling a little better and went to type a text on my phone, I thought, *Oh, they're* not *all tigers!* The dancing lady was still just a dancing lady and not a dancing tiger in a red dress.

At least it was something I could look back and laugh about. There was zero other laughter coming out of that day. Just bad news that was hard to take lightly.

As I was getting discharged from the hospital, I was pretty nervous sitting in the wheelchair. Yes, I was happy to go home, but what if I didn't know how to manage my drains? What if I screwed up? Should I get a night nurse? I didn't know up from down.

When we did leave, I had John drive *very* slowly. He went over a speed bump at one point and I almost filed for divorce. Someone had told me to place a pillow between myself and the seatbelt, which helped tremendously, but it was still agony riding in the car.

When we arrived home, the house was filled with flowers. I was overcome with emotion because never in my wildest dreams did I expect so many people to think of me. Maybe I would have expected a bouquet or two, and a few notes, but this was really beyond. I'd never seen so many arrangements in one room—it took my breath away. And because I am who I am and *cannot* help myself, I immediately walked in and started rearranging the flowers. That arrangement certainly didn't belong next to that arrangement, and what about color order! I had to get to work.

My mother yelled, "Clea! Stop it. Sit down."

"Mom, I can't! The lilies are on the table! They should be on the counter."

"Well, then, I guess you're feeling okay," she said and laughed, seemingly relieved. "But still: Sit down and stop it right now." She also added her favorite phrase, one I have heard one million times before: "Clea, I am your *mother*."

Yikes. It was like using my middle name except that she had never given me one (a story for another time, but let's just say I *thought* my middle name was Lynn until I was twenty-one years old, at which point the Social Security Administration informed me otherwise). This was code for "Listen to me right now and do as I say." Fair enough. I did feel like I could handle some flower organization, but the day before I'd thought all the emojis were tiger faces, so maybe I wasn't trustworthy in this department.

One day after my surgery, I felt well enough to walk around the house, albeit slowly. I felt pretty confident at that point that I could stop taking strong pain medication. Given all the stories in the news about opioid addiction, I had a justified fear of opioids, and I didn't want to take the OxyContin that had been prescribed. I actually had a moment when I tried to make a grandiose statement about not needing the Oxy—I marched to the toilet to flush them down the drain. But we had put in these fancy toilets that flush automatically and they weren't working properly. So now I just had a pile of OxyContin sitting in my toilet and bubbling while they slowly dissolved.

I wasn't worried about getting rid of the Oxy (once it was actually flushed down the toilet) because I had a host of other medications to take that would hopefully make me comfortable enough. Fingers crossed for the ultra-strength ibuprofen and Tylenol!

Was I in pain? Of course. But was it manageable? Honestly, yes. And I am a very, very delicate flower. The most pain I had encountered until that point was wisdom teeth extraction at age sixteen. Do not picture me getting a cartilage ear piercing or, heaven forbid, a tattoo. I am *not* tough when it comes to pain, but remarkably, recovery from this surgery was something I could handle.

My plastic surgeon had asked John to take progress photos of my breasts as the days went on so he could monitor how I was healing. Obviously, the surgery hadn't gone as planned, and we still needed to keep things under a microscope while the dust settled. I have to admit, I never looked at what was underneath the bandages because I was too afraid of what I might see. I let John be my eyes so I could dismiss my fears and not have to look. I was encased in bandages that needed to be changed, with drains that needed to be emptied.

"Drain" may sound weird, but it's just a tube taking fluid away from the surgical area and into a bulb that can be emptied. A quick PSA for drains: I was pretty scared by their reputation, but it wasn't that bad. They don't hurt, they're just annoying and one more thing to deal with. They sound very intimidating, but they're really nothing to worry about.

As soon as Dr. Perdikis began receiving the photos he became concerned. John tried to sugarcoat this a bit for me, but it was hard to conceal that something had to be done immediately. My skin was starting to turn black—a sign of necrosis. You hear about these things being a possibility, but it's rare.

Dr. Perdikis prescribed me a cream that John would have to apply twice daily. The hope was that it would draw blood back to the dying cells and bring them back to life. More praise for John because if I had to do it myself, I would have been like, *Nah, I'm good*. He got to work applying this cream while changing my bandages and emptying my drains, all while continuing to send Dr. Perdikis daily photo updates. This cream, ironically, caused more pain than my actual surgery. It triggered horrific headaches that I found myself taking medication for. And ultimately it did not work.

My doctor spelled things out for me in no uncertain terms: A swift operation for the necrosis was needed. If we waited, he couldn't guarantee a good outcome. About a week after my double mastectomy, on Easter Sunday, Dr. Meszoely showed up to the hospital with an amaryllis plant as an Easter gift. When Dr. Perdikis saw this reminder of the holiday, he apologized for the bad timing.

"Don't worry, I'm Jewish," I said. "Let's do this."

Dr. Perdikis wanted to brace me for the possibility that the surgery wouldn't work. There was a chance I would have to remain flat-chested if they couldn't get this corrected. My skin was in a pretty dire place, and while I hadn't seen it for myself, I could tell the severity of the situation. I had to remind myself, again, about the need to pivot based on new information, and to have faith in the new plan presented to me. Also, let's be real, what choice did I have?

What I didn't realize at the time, which my doctor told me later, was that how quickly I agreed to have that second surgery was what saved my entire situation. My willingness to pivot in a new direction made all the difference.

"Most people would be gun-shy about going back in," Dr. Perdikis said, "or they'd want to think about various options. They'd want to take their time to consider. Because you acted so decisively, I think [it] made the difference in us getting a result we could work with."

I was glad to find that out, and relieved that I had acted without hesitation. But I had also started to realize that along my journey, there would be more of this—more critical moments, more pivots, more urgency. I was *not* a fan of twists and turns, and I needed to buckle up, because there would be many more.

One Thing

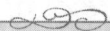

Cancer is complicated not just for the person receiving treatment. It's a challenge for the whole household, particularly a spouse or partner. Something that John experienced was wondering how to navigate his life and his career as a photographer outside my cancer journey. Whether it was at work or a social event, he found even simple conversations difficult. He would run into clients, friends, or acquaintances at photo shoots or work events, and when they'd engage in normal banter like, "How's the family?" his mind would jump immediately to *Does this person know what we've been through this year? Do I tell them? Should I say the family is well, or do I say Clea has cancer?*

When he decided to answer the question honestly and frankly, he felt like it detonated a bomb. So he ended up trying to avoid these interactions as much as possible, which started to take a toll on his well-being. The best remedy was for John to have his own network of friends he could talk to. Spouses of patients, survivors, and his inner circle became his lifeline. A note to all partners: Remember that you need to be cared for too. There is a lot to navigate during treatment and beyond. Having a support system is paramount.

CHAPTER TEN

The Red Devil

With my second surgery behind me, and my doctors confident that I was on the road to recovery from my double mastectomy, it felt like I could finally start to move forward and make progress in my recovery.

One of the things that helped me during this time (and something that I always share with anyone who is going through any surgery or treatment that will limit mobility) is renting a medical recliner. This dark brown leather chair could move me from a flat, horizontal position to a standing position with the click of a remote. Let me tell you, that recliner was a lifesaver. Is it cool looking? Absolutely not. Is it *the* most game-changing solution? Yes. Some nights I even slept in it. I positioned it in the living room because I didn't want to be isolated in the bedroom. I wanted to feel the movement of the house and be a participant in my family's life, to have everyone and everything going on around me. I didn't want to be sequestered in a separate space where depression might lurk.

And for physical comfort too—wow, did I need that chair. When you get a double mastectomy, all the movements involving your chest are severely limited because the pain is so intense. And you don't even realize which motions will trigger those nerves until it's too late. The searing pain that shot through me when I pressed the volume button on my phone, for instance, shocked me. The chair helped alleviate some of this because I could recline without needing to pull myself up to a sitting position. It could also help me stand up. That chair—five stars, would recommend.

My mother, though, proved even more useful than the chair throughout those weeks. John was my caregiver, bandage changer, drain operator, parent in chief, and all-around saint. But my mom was my cheerleader, laugh partner, and overall comfort blanket. As an adult, I have never needed my mother as much as I did at that time. I didn't anticipate how much it would soothe me, but the second I got sick, I instinctively wanted my mother. And as most moms do, she also deployed some tough love (John would *never*). For one thing, she made me go on a walk every day even if I insisted that I was too tired. I mean, she wouldn't let me organize flowers—can't I even nap? No, it was time to get up and get our steps in.

The first day we just walked to the stop sign at the end of the street. The next day we went a full block. Pretty soon, a few weeks had passed and we were doing two miles. In my mind, I might as well have won an Olympic medal. I posted a photo to Instagram from one of the days when I didn't think I was going to be able to make it very far, but I kept going—in my pajama top, no less. Eventually, I made it back home and was filled with such pride.

I could actually do this! Here I was, after a major surgery, and I was stronger than I ever knew.

But there was also another feeling creeping in during that period.

Every day I got better, I knew I was moving closer to the next phase of treatment. I wanted to celebrate each passing day and how well I was recovering, but that optimism was mixed with anxiety and fear of what was to come.

I was still living in my post-surgery bubble, suspended in a recovery period that I didn't want to end. Those were the few precious weeks when I improved each day rather than getting weaker. I was still able to check in with work (I was technically taking time off, but some habits die hard) and have lengthy conversations with Joanna to get updates. I was able to go on a road trip to the beach with John and the kids. It was freezing, but we knew it was our last trip before chemo started. I was able to go to lunch with friends, or have them come visit at the house, without becoming exhausted. All in all, I was enjoying a slice of normalcy, and I wasn't ready for it to end.

I knew it was time to wrap my head around part two of this journey. Dr. Park, my oncologist, was due to call any minute—this would be the moment of truth. I thought back to a few weeks earlier when there was a possibility I wouldn't even *need* chemo. Those hopes had been dashed following the discovery of cancer in my lymph nodes, but because I didn't know my course of treatment yet, I was still holding out hope that it wouldn't include chemo.

When Dr. Park called at the end of April, he emphasized that he wanted me to recover more before we moved to next steps, but he wanted to prepare me for what was ahead.

"I know I'm going to need chemo," I said.

He paused. Then he said, "Unfortunately, in your case, it is going to be necessary."

He laid out the plans.

In my case, there were going to be four rounds, over the course of eight weeks, of the dreaded red devil. Each round would be delivered via intravenous infusions through a port that would soon be placed in my chest. The red devil was the drug Lauren B. had warned me about. Its proper name is AC: Adriamycin and cyclophosphamide. It's a common drug combination for battling breast cancer, but that didn't make it any more palatable.

Following AC, I would need twelve rounds over twelve weeks of Taxol, a different cancer-fighting drug. I looked it up and saw that it wasn't supposed to make you as sick as the red devil, which was undeniably going to be brutal. AC has to be administered every other week because your body needs time to recover between doses. Taxol is more easily tolerated and can be done weekly.

After eight weeks of the red devil and twelve weeks of Taxol, I would move on to six weeks of radiation: five days a week for six weeks.

Dr. Park explained that at my age (forty at the time), it was important that I receive a full course of treatment. They were going to throw the kitchen sink at me. He reminded me my cancer was curable, and I had a long life to live. And because I was relatively young, it was possible I would weather chemotherapy with relative ease. I agreed with and understood everything he was saying, but it didn't stop the absolute flood of tears.

Having this conversation with my oncologist was the second time in my cancer journey when I found myself uncontrollably crying, the first being the original diagnosis. I didn't cry after either of the surgeries and I didn't cry during the recovery. But hearing my chemotherapy and radiation treatment laid out made me lose it.

I pelted Dr. Park (he is going to be so annoyed I haven't called him Ben for so many chapters) with questions:

"Will I have any quality of life?"

"How bad will I feel?"

"Will I be physically sick all the time?"

His answers were very measured. It's hard to predict how an individual will respond to treatment, but he had high hopes I would do well.

I'd never heard of a single person—no matter how young or healthy—come out of chemotherapy with a positive review. Zero people said AC was totally cool and there was no need to worry.

Part of the reason I wanted to name this book *Cancer Is Complicated* is because of the range of emotions I experienced day-to-day and week-to-week. I didn't cry every day—far from it. There were a lot of days when I was just experiencing important, wonderful, and meaningful moments. And then there were others, like that phone call about my chemo treatment, when everything imploded. But thankfully, these implosions were few and far between.

In the days that followed, there was a weird juxtaposition of feeling better and stronger, while also knowing that I was just marching toward a different battle. I envisioned all the people who were able to enjoy their recovery because they didn't have to endure the chemotherapy that followed. I had pangs of jealousy because that had *almost* been me. I had gotten a taste of thinking that would be my path, and then poof, that dream was gone.

Since Paris, I had been committed to not feeling sorry for myself. I didn't believe in self-pity, and I certainly didn't believe in wallowing. But when I thought about my chemo plan, it was hard to keep feelings of sadness and fear from popping into my head. Chemo scared me more than cancer. I was so fearful and so overwhelmed. If you're just about to start chemo and scared as hell right now, I want to say this: I was too. In fact, I don't know a single patient who wasn't. But we're all here standing on the other side.

Another thing I don't like to indulge in is regret. You live and learn. I've made a million mistakes in my life, and I regret zero of them because they all led to important lessons. There's no point in wasting time with what would, could, or should have been. But I would find myself thinking I *could have* prevented the cancer spreading to my lymph nodes had I taken self-exams more seriously. If I had allowed it to sink in that very first time I felt something, in July 2021, rather than dismissing it entirely. What if I had listened to my body? Could I have changed the course of my entire life? The answer is most definitely yes. But like I said, every mistake has led to learning, and I very much hope I pass that learning forward.

With this in mind, I'd force myself to snap back to reality and accept that I had been dealt a blow I would never forget. And I vowed to scream it from the rooftops so that others wouldn't make the same mistake I did. I needed to dust myself off and push forward, put my armor back on, and prepare to fight like my life depended on it. Because it did.

One Thing

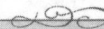

Things I Recommend Following Surgery

- Medical recliner chair (just search for local chair rentals)
- Magnesium citrate or milk of magnesia (in case the anesthesia or various medications cause constipation)
- Zip-up sweatshirt with interior pockets for drains (if you have them)
- Pajamas and shirts that button in front
- Bras that zip in the front (I prefer zip rather than hook-and-eye closures)
- Book you can't put down (this is not the time for a long autobiography—get yourself a mystery or thriller)
- Watch list of TV series or movies (poll your friends for suggestions)
- Favorite snacks
- Cozy blanket
- Anything that brings you comfort (candle, framed photo, flowers)

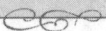

CHAPTER ELEVEN

Preparations

I want to say again how much my mother helped me keep going, especially when I was scared, transitioning from post-surgery into chemotherapy. She stayed with John and me for almost my entire surgery recovery and would only take time off to see my dad for a week, before traveling back to be with me for another five weeks. She would continue that way—five weeks with us, one week at home—through my entire course of treatment. She was there for me through everything. Not since having the chicken pox as a child had I received such attentive care.

Because I was recovering nicely from surgery, and before chemotherapy was set to begin, my mother was leaving for the first time to go home. We gave each other a big hug, and then she looked at me, laughing through her tears, put her hands on my shoulders, and said, "But didn't we have so much fun?"

We both cried and laughed because it was *true*! Against all odds, we were having a great time being together while I recovered from surgery. How on earth were we *enjoying* this time together? How many chances do you get as an adult to spend so much quality time with your mother? I wasn't distracted with work or social plans, so we really just got to . . . hang out. It was a time filled with so much love, and the sadness was kept at a distance. Again, cancer is complicated. There are so many cherished moments alongside the difficult ones. In my journey, there would be plenty of both.

While my mother was staying with us, we developed this routine with John (and my dad when he would come visit): Every night, once the kids were in bed, we would watch two episodes of whatever TV series we had landed on. Sometimes I laugh when I think about it, because for some reason, we ended up in a period of TV that included shows starring Toni Collette (*Pieces of Her* and *The Staircase*) and series about female con artists (*Inventing Anna*, *The Dropout*, and *Bad Vegan*). Of all the things to remember during my cancer journey, this TV marathon will go down in my mental history.

Trigger alert: In *Pieces of Me*, Toni Collette is actually playing a character with cancer who is going through chemotherapy. You don't realize just how many shows and movies involve cancer as part of the plot until cancer is part of your plot too. You start watching something, and after you're halfway through, there it is—a main character, a friend, or a parent, sick with cancer or dying from cancer.

I'd like to have a word with Hollywood and ask them to maybe stop. We should also stop implying that a horrible outcome is a given. Not everyone's experience will involve dark, gloomy rooms with metal chairs lined up in a row and end in death. I actually think they use a gray filter in these scenes to make it look as depressing as possible. Cancer is depressing enough! Does it need to look like it's taking place inside a storm cloud? The gloomy cancer plots became so egregious that I started researching shows and movies beforehand to make sure I wouldn't step into the same trap over and over. I was about to head into chemo, and these shows were not helping my outlook.

The week before chemo was supposed to start, in mid-May, Joanna and I filmed video content for a branded campaign we were working on. I was so anxious because this was my first attempt at going back to in-person work post-surgery. I didn't realize that I was supposed to try on multiple outfits for the shoot.

I was handed the first shirt to try on and started to put it on, but I couldn't.

Searing pain shot through my whole body.

I burst into tears on set and had to go into another room. I was ashamed to admit it, but I had to walk out of the dressing area wearing the same thing I'd arrived in. *I couldn't even pull a shirt over my head yet.*

I felt like my body was broken and wouldn't be coming back anytime soon. I'm not a person who does well with giving less than 100 percent, and I couldn't even put a shirt on. Here I was, about to start this seemingly horrific treatment, and my body was still so thoroughly compromised. I was used to the difficulty it caused at home, but I hadn't yet reckoned with this at work. This would be the third time that I sobbed, this time out of frustration with my physical limitations and lack of mobility.

I had a lot of private moments of frustration, sadness, and anger, but this was one of the most real moments, when I just wanted to scream out loud at cancer. Joanna was with me that day on the set and full of compassion for what I was going through. She had a few choice words for cancer herself.

She hugged me as tight as she could without hurting me.

"You have every right to cry," she said. "We can just sit on the floor and cry as long as you want."

The crew figured out pain-free fashion choices for me, for which I was grateful, albeit embarrassed. I was able to collect myself, finish the shoot, and drive back home. But I did call John from the car to cry a little bit more because my emotions continued to hit me minute by minute.

Over the next few days, we tried to focus on having all the essentials for chemo together before things got underway. I received *so* many thoughtful things from friends, loved ones, and work associates. From cozy socks to crystals, and from special lotions to good luck charms, much of it helped me greatly. I will always be so grateful to those who were generous with their love, their thoughtfulness, their kindness . . . it meant the world.

One Thing

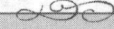

My Personal Watch List During Treatment

- *Succession*
- *Top Chef*
- *The White Lotus*
- *Stranger Things*
- *The Patient*
- *Only Murders in the Building*
- *Surface*
- *The Watcher*
- *Painkiller* (This one really makes you want to lean on ibuprofen!)
- *Daisy Jones and the Six*

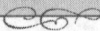

One More Thing

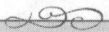

Chemo Essentials

(If you're looking to give a gift or you get asked for a chemo wish list, here are some ideas!)

- Barefoot Dreams anything (robe, blanket, socks)
- An e-reader (I don't leave home without one, and it makes reading during chemo and other appointments so easy)
- Personalized tote bag to bring on chemo days
- Good luck charms (I received everything from a silver four-leaf clover to a little gold Buddha)
- Comfortable and lightweight pajamas (regulating body temperature can be hard)
- A care package with a reusable water bottle, favorite snacks, and a candle
- A donation to breast cancer research

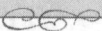

CHAPTER TWELVE

Here Comes Chemo

I was scheduled to receive chemotherapy at the Vanderbilt-Ingram Cancer Center in Nashville. When I walked in for my first round on May 19, I was absolutely terrified. I clutched my tote bag of suggested essentials—heated blankets, water, Diet Coke (don't fight me, my life was hard enough), my Kindle, and my cell phone—and walked back to the infusion room. I resisted the urge to interview people in the other rooms to get their hot takes on chemo; I assumed their reviews would be not great. My kids had given me cards, and I laughed out loud when I read "I hope chemo doesn't make you emo."

Thank goodness for some levity; I'm someone who needs that.

I learned that my sessions would each last a couple of hours, so we had some time to fill while we were there. Between the pre-meds, the anti-nausea medication, icing my port, the actual infusion, and flushing my port at the end, it's a fairly lengthy regimen. John, my mom, and I all found our own ways to pass the time. John would bring his computer to get work done. (He took off as much time as possible, but he still had to make priority shoots happen.) My mother packed a bag of needlepoint supplies. (During my entire course of treatment she was working on an elaborate Christmas stocking for Sutton. She has needlepointed one for each of us even though, as I mentioned, we are Jewish. Her need to craft outweighs religion.)

Each patient in the facility had their own private space with three walls and a curtain instead of a door. This allowed us to spread out and be as comfortable as three people could be given the circumstances. The nurses (true MVPs) would then come around with a box of snacks. I always picked the Fritos. Not exactly the healthiest option, but the heart wants what the heart wants.

The first phase of my chemotherapy started with four rounds of AC (hello there, red devil!) over the course of eight weeks (one session every other week). In this first phase, all these treatments would follow a similar pattern.

I would receive AC on Thursday and feel fine. On Friday I would feel not great, but not terrible. I would spend Saturday pretty sick (mostly nausea and fatigue, but also bone pain, hot flashes, and a variety of pains that can only be described as WTF is that?), sipping on ginger ale and eating saltines. By Sunday I would start to rebound and the worst was over. For the next ten days, I'd feel fine. Then I'd go in for another round. I started to believe, and hope, and feel confident that throughout treatment I was going to have more good days than bad days.

Shout-out to the staff at Vanderbilt-Ingram: Everyone went out of their way to make each patient feel so cared for. It never felt like a sad day walking into the office, which was pretty surprising given that I was there for something that was objectively pretty sad.

Among the other items that helped make chemo a lot easier: my chemo port. During my necrosis surgery I had a port placed in my upper chest. That would mean I could avoid constant needles in my veins; the port provided all the access necessary. The nurses would simply numb the area and then inject the drugs directly into my port. It was strange living with the port at first. You could see the little lump protruding from my skin, and it felt weird to the touch because it's very obviously a foreign object. On the other hand, it felt like a badge of honor, always reminding me what was at stake.

I had a *lot* of questions for the nurses in those early days: Would I get sick immediately? Would I feel the drugs entering my system? How often was I allowed to take Zofran for nausea? Was it time yet for my antianxiety med, Ativan? If I was lucky (and if the nurses were luckier), I would get enough answers quickly so I could nod off.

But there was no sleeping through my first round! That first time, I remained wide awake and hyperaware of everything.

The first sensation I had: gratitude for how hard the staff clearly worked to make patients cozy. I was extremely fortunate that I got to sit in a comfortable room in a reclining chair with heat settings. The nurses brought me blankets to help with the chill. At that point I noticed that I'd been shivering. I wondered: *Am I freezing or just shaking from nerves?*

The first dose of medication had to be hand-administered by a nurse instead of a machine. Somehow that was comforting to me. It was like having adult supervision. As the drugs began to flow through the tubes, it was a shocking bright red. I didn't realize the red devil was in fact red in color. I broke into a laugh when I realized the shirt I had selected, with zippered access to my port, was also bright red. For whatever reason, that took the edge off and made the moment less somber.

I looked around the room at my surroundings to distract myself. John was in one chair working on his computer and my mother was in another chair needlepointing. And I was in *my* chair, white-knuckled and worried. In addition to the TV on the wall, I had brought my Kindle, my phone, and loads of snacks. I didn't feel up for any of it so I just stared into space. But pretty soon it was over, and I didn't feel any different. Not yet, at least.

As the red devil began entering my body that first day, it felt more mentally taxing in the moment than physically taxing. There was something about it that felt surreal to me, to see the medication flowing directly into my body. This was the moment everyone talks about. It was starting, and there were no backsies.

When it was over, it took me a minute to realize that I was finished. Round one was done! I went into my mental checklist and crossed off the first round. It had only just ended, but now I was 25 percent done with AC, and I wanted to celebrate the achievement. My second thought was that my body was now a science experiment, and I had no idea how or when it would react to the drugs in my system. I wanted to go home and sit in my recliner and wait for something to happen. It turned out I could take a beat from infusion day, because the side effects didn't start to kick in until the day after. That's when I started tracking which were going to be my good days and which would be my bad days.

It sounds trivial in the grand scheme of things, but one of my absolute biggest fears with cancer was throwing up. I have a terrible phobia of vomiting (it's actually called emetophobia), and I hadn't thrown up since I was ten years old. I know how silly this sounds when you're fighting for your life, but it was potentially my biggest fear. One of the most widely known side effects of chemotherapy is, of course, nausea and vomiting. We've all seen it depicted in every commercial, show, and movie involving a cancer patient. Thank you once again, Hollywood, for continuing to freak me out. I asked my doctor if it was possible not to throw up during the course of treatment, and Dr. Park said very assuredly that it was absolutely possible with the help of the provided medications.

Oh, he had yet to see my dedication to this cause.

For the few days following my first chemo infusion, I would alternate between the anti-nausea meds Zofran and Compazine around the clock. It's kind of like alternating between Advil and Tylenol so that you always had something working in your favor. When one drug was halfway through, the other would be starting. To this day, I have not thrown up from cancer treatment even once. Was I sick to my stomach and did I have debilitating nausea at times? Of course. Did I lie on the bathroom floor more than once? Yes. But I managed to control this one aspect of this illness, and that made a big difference. There's so much you *can't* control with cancer, so I believed in controlling the controllables whenever possible.

Staying organized with all the information I was collecting also gave me a brief semblance of control over my situation. That's another suggestion I have for anyone going through this: Keep a notebook in which you track your symptoms and treatments. And let's be real, in my case when I say notebook I mean the Notes app on my phone. But whatever works for you, use it!

I doubt it will come as a shock to you that I was desperate to learn every single, solitary thing I could about what was to come. That's where my collective of breast cancer friends came in. I had reached out to my close friends who had experienced breast cancer in the past, including Christina Applegate, my two Laurens, and Stevie. They got me through those very early days. My dear friend Christina was my absolute rock from day one of my diagnosis. Since her own journey with breast cancer, she's been a longtime outspoken advocate for early detection and prevention. Christina was a wealth of information, and she spent hours on the phone with me—and even with John while I was in surgery. But soon, I had friends connecting me with their friends, and my team started to grow.

I began to accumulate an even wider circle through everyone's goodwill: a friend's coworker, someone's cousin, a friend of a friend of a friend. I gladly would talk to anyone who would talk to me. Some had already been through cancer, some were currently in treatment, and some had just been diagnosed. We would check in, commiserate, ask questions, send photos and updates. These women became my lifeline.

When I'd been in Paris right after my diagnosis, I would spend hours on the phone with different people, often during the middle of the night my time. I needed to hear their stories in order to understand what my own would be. I needed to hear that my life wasn't going to be over. I would hold on tight to their stories of battling and beating cancer and making it to the other side. I could be like them, I thought. That was my first experience creating these connections, and it was so powerful. Talking to these women changed the course of my life because it gave me hope when I felt extremely hopeless. I knew that my relationships with them would be the way I could endure this period of my life.

Some of these women who I have spent an inordinate amount of time with via text and phone I have still not met to this day. My friend Lori (who I was introduced to by my friend Maria) and I had a nearly identical treatment plan—we spoke multiple times each day—and we have still never met. It's wild to have such a close and intimate friendship, in which you share photos of yourself scarred, sick, and bald, and you know the gory details of every ailment, but not, for instance, where they grew up or how they met their husband. One thing I remember vividly, though, is how anxious Lori was about her survival. Like I said before, I had a million fears, but not surviving wasn't one of them. It just goes to show how two people going through the exact same thing can have two different approaches to the disease.

Lori lives in Seattle and is still healthy and thriving. I need to get out there eventually so I can give her a hug in person and compare our hair length. We even talk about planning a survivors' trip to somewhere fabulous. (We really need to get on that.) But others I *have* been lucky to meet, and each time it's been like encountering a long-lost friend.

One of those friends was Maria (who I was introduced to by a friend in L.A., and then Maria connected me to Lori—I know it's confusing! Bear with me). Maria had beaten breast cancer *twice*. And in her twenties, no less! Just a reminder that cancer doesn't care how old you are. It was always so helpful to get Maria's point of view on everything because she had already lived through it. I would text Lori about what she was going through *now*, but I could text Maria about what she went through *then*. It was also a bonus that she made me laugh. It's of course a somber time, and not everyone is up for laughing with you. Find yourself a friend who can find the humor in things, because it helps.

Over the summer, during chemo, the *Today* show asked if I could provide an on-air health update and bring in a couple of my new cancer friends, who I could meet in person for the first time. When Maria and Amy (a friend of a friend from Nashville) walked onto the set, I got so emotional! I had been texting with these women *so* much—sometimes hours each day—and here they were! Like I mentioned, Maria had already beaten cancer, but Amy and I were in the thick of it. She was one of my lifelines. I just couldn't get over the fact that I could hug them for the first time and say thank you for being beside me. Also I was shocked that they were both so much taller than me. Might have been nice to get a heels memo, ladies.

While we were taping the show, Hoda asked us each about our calming and happiest spot during treatment. For her, it had been walking in Central Park. For me, it was sitting in my usual chair on my back porch in Nashville. For Maria, it had been sitting on the beach (she is the beachiest beach babe you've ever seen) in L.A. And for Amy, it was a bench she would walk to by the water in Hoboken. All of us needed shelter from the storm that had entered our lives, and it gave me solace to think about friends and strangers alike, all experiencing the same sense of comfort.

There was another friend, Leslie, who I spoke to extensively in the early days, and she continued to help me all the way through treatment. Leslie and I are mutual friends of yet another Lauren— Lauren C. Lauren C. had introduced me to Leslie the minute she heard about my diagnosis. Leslie, having been through this before, so generously took my midnight panic phone calls from Paris right after my diagnosis. To say I was losing my mind on that trip would have been an understatement, and Leslie talked me off the ledge more than a few times.

Leslie had already been through treatment, so she gave me a detailed explanation of how her days, weeks, and months had felt, and how she could even go from a sick Sunday afternoon to playing tennis with Lauren on Tuesday. I don't play tennis even on my healthiest days with perfect weather conditions, but it was reassuring to know that I *could*. Also, the outfits are very chic. If I had to pick up a sport, it would be tennis. I think I actually promised to play with them when I was finally well. And Laguna Beach is a quick drive from L.A., so I guessed I'd better figure out how to swing a racket.

Collecting these strong, insightful, kind, honest women in my life motivated me to be the same for them and, one day, for someone else. From what I understand, this is pretty common in breast cancer communities. If someone needs help, has questions, needs someone—to cry with, laugh with, scream with, confide with—your tribe will rise to the occasion.

Hearing everyone else's stories and experiences also made me realize we had one thing in common: We were all here to tell the tale. We were all alive and not going anywhere. These were the nuggets of hope that I hung on to, even as I was bracing myself for the worst.

One Thing

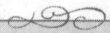

Your cancer community circle is truly your lifeline. Let your friends and network connect you to people you've never met, and hold on to them for dear life. Some of my closest relationships today are with women I met via text. To cultivate your circle, I recommend having a mix of people who have already experienced breast cancer treatment (in all forms—not everyone had to have chemo or the same course of treatment) and people who are going through treatment alongside you. It is *so* helpful to be able to ask questions of someone who has already been through it, and it is equally helpful to ask the people in your position what they are experiencing. Cultivating a community is key and will make all the difference.

I started to immediately be connected with people when I posted publicly on social media that I had been diagnosed and was about to undergo a double mastectomy. I had the good fortune (and still do!) to have a platform that accelerated the development of my new community, but there are plenty of alternatives to find connections in other ways. The best option is, of course, through friends and family introductions. It's a more personal network, and it's always nice to have someone in common.

The sad reality is that most of us have at least one person in our lives who has battled breast cancer, or another type of cancer, so these connections are fairly easy to make. But if you *don't* have much of a personal network, start with the cancer center where you are receiving treatment. There is usually a support group you can access if you talk to your doctor or nurses.

No matter how you collect your network, don't be afraid to reach out. Often. Survivors are usually grateful to have the opportunity to counsel others and answer questions, and patients who are experiencing treatment are often happy to have another person to talk with, share notes, and lean on.

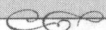

CHAPTER THIRTEEN

Taking Back Control

The Vanderbilt-Ingram Cancer Center sat near one of my family's favorite restaurants, Bistro 360, so we developed a routine of going there after each infusion (apologies for always being in pajamas at this very lovely establishment). I would have a nice champagne lunch with my mom and John, and then I would take an afternoon nap. Not a bad day, all things considered.

That first round of chemo was manageable, but after that things started to get dicey. Chemotherapy is cumulative, so it builds in your system over time—meaning you will likely feel exponentially worse with each infusion. So the way you feel the first time will not be the way you feel every time. In a weird way, it was sort of like being pregnant—you start having all these symptoms at the beginning of the process, but you don't know how they will progress.

At the start of chemotherapy, I mostly experienced nausea and fatigue. I took a lot of Zofran that first time because I was determined not to throw up, but I knew there was another side effect coming up, and it wasn't sickness. I was about to start losing my hair.

I went back to my mantra about controlling the controllables, and I decided to shave off my hair before the second round of chemo, when it might start to fall out on its own. If I was going to lose my hair, it was going to be on my terms. For my own mental health, I framed it as an emotional milestone instead of a painful event. I had my makeup done that day so John could take a photo of me that I felt good about. I had my friends there to hold my hand, I had my mom. . . . I was as ready as I would ever be. But no matter how much I prepared myself, I couldn't help but completely break down when I saw my bare head in the mirror. This wasn't a moment of vanity. It felt more like a limb had been sawed off. And considering I was still recovering from my double mastectomy—in which I did have actual body parts taken off—it was tough not to feel like all my femininity had been taken from me.

As I started to adjust to my new appearance, I found myself, in equal parts, feeling empowered by my choice and embarrassed about what I looked like. Would my husband still be attracted to me? Would my kids be embarrassed to be in public with me—or even be uncomfortable in private with me? I tried to get a grip. This was just hair. But why did it feel like so much more than that?

It turned out hair is more important than one would think. I realized that without it I finally looked sick. I looked like a textbook cancer patient. After my surgery, I was just bandaged up—I didn't look like I had cancer. Now that I didn't have hair, it was a neon sign flashing to anyone and everyone. And it wasn't just a flashing sign to them; it was a flashing sign to me.

There are actually a lot of options for people to keep their hair, I just didn't choose them. You can cold cap, which involves icing your scalp during chemo. That isn't always effective, and I honestly didn't feel strong enough to handle one more variable. I had decided that my emotions and stress level needed to be managed more than my physical appearance. This might not be the best choice for everyone out there. I had plenty of friends choose to cold cap and try to preserve their hair. But I didn't have it in me.

Breast cancer strips you of so much dignity. I never considered myself to be a vain person. I'm average height, thin-ish, with a small cup size, and I wore hair extensions because my natural hair was mediocre. I didn't feel particularly attached to the way I looked, to be honest. But losing my hair and my breasts made me feel untethered to my own body in ways I didn't expect. Once my hair was shaved and the bandages were off, I had to face what I looked like and how much I had changed. I waited until the day before chemo to look at my breasts.

I had been healing for six weeks and I was too afraid to look that whole time. John, meanwhile, had been looking twice a day, and I figured if I looked like Frankenstein, he would tell me. (I don't know why I ever assumed that. When I thought about it, John would rather move to another country in the middle of the night than tell me I looked anything other than beautiful.) John was the one who changed my bandages and my drains and put on ointment. He was with me at every single doctor visit and witnessed the realest of the real. If anyone could bear it, it was John.

So, I looked for the first time. I stood there topless, looking into the full-length mirror, and I was shocked by what I saw. To my eyes, I looked like a bald, bloated, flat-chested man.

It was hard to acknowledge that I actually cared about appearance when I was fighting for my life. But the reflection staring back at me in the mirror was less like myself and more like Harry Goldenblatt, Charlotte's husband in *Sex and the City*.

I know that sounds silly, but it's hard to have confidence when the person you see looking back at you is such a warped version of how you see yourself. It's hard to have any self-esteem when that person is absent any markers of what we've been taught signifies beauty.

I tried wigs at first when I was fully bald. I did it mainly because I thought baldness made *other* people uncomfortable. It's uncomfortable not only for those of us experiencing it but also for those around us. No one knows exactly what to say or how to act. And maybe most important, I didn't want my children to feel ashamed to be out with me in public. But the second I had even the smallest amount of fuzz on my head, something like a fresh peach, I acted as if I had a full head of hair. I ditched the scarves and the wigs and decided to finally accept my appearance once and for all. Not to mention it was the middle of summer in Tennessee, and I wasn't going to beat cancer just to die from heatstroke.

Another reason I had decided to shave my head was because I had made a personal commitment to be outspoken and vocal about my very real journey. I hoped that maybe by choosing this for myself, I could help other women feel empowered while going through something similar. That they might feel like they could take matters into their own hands as well. I wanted people to feel less afraid. *I* wanted to feel less afraid. I was determined to get a grip on my own sorrow so that I could make that a reality.

One Thing

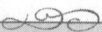

There are so many different approaches to hair when undergoing chemo treatment. You can let your hair fall out, you can shave it off, you can try to hang on to it with cold capping. And if you opt for a wig, there is also a wide variety of choices out there.

In my case, I had a couple of wigs made with real hair and styled to match my hair pre-cancer. These kinds of wigs can be pricey but can also be styled with heat tools because the hair is real. I also went to a wig shop and purchased a couple of synthetic wigs that come pre-styled. Synthetic wigs are very easy to pop on and much more affordable.

Here are some things to consider when shopping for a wig:

- Do your research on local wig shops and online resources (I used both Google and Instagram) to view all your options.

- Do you have a budget in mind? Custom wigs can be very costly, and wigs made with real hair are quite expensive. If you prefer a more affordable option, synthetic is the way to go.

- Do you want to spend the time to wash and style your wig? Real hair means real effort, which is time-consuming.

- Do you want wigs in various hairstyles? You can get a few pre-styled options to mix it up!

- Before buying multiple wigs, consider where and how you will store them. I bought Styrofoam wig heads online and added a floating shelf in my closet.

Yet another option, and one that works surprisingly well, are baseball hats that have hair sewn in. The hair doesn't cover the top, just the sides, so it's a nice option for hot weather. Both the hair and the hats come in all sorts of colors and styles.

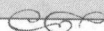

CHAPTER FOURTEEN

"Mommy, You're Beautiful"

My kids knew what was going to be happening with my hair, with my body. I had warned them. I was worried that they were going to say something that could unintentionally sting, just because that's how kids can be. I also worried about what other kids might say to them. Having their mom sick with cancer was hard enough. Kids can be so cruel, and I was worried about their friends making fun of them for having a mother who looked like . . . me.

I cared a lot less about my personal struggles than I did about how my kids were going to process their own. When I was younger, I used to be upset when my mom wore the wrong kind of jeans. I couldn't imagine how I would've felt if she'd started walking around bald.

Like I said, it took me a while initially to tell my children I had cancer. At the time, both Stella and Sutton seemed to understand what was happening and they both had the same question: "Are you going to lose your hair?"

It was a fair question. Because there's sick, and then there's lose-your-hair sick. There's sick, and then there's chemo-sick. Even at their young ages they knew the difference.

When I first told them, I'd thought I might not need chemo because the cancer cells hadn't spread into my lymph nodes. I replied honestly when I told them I didn't think I needed to lose my hair. Radiation, however, was a given, but maybe I could just do that in conjunction with my ongoing hormone therapy.

For anyone who doesn't know the difference—which I also didn't—chemo attacks your whole body, whereas radiation is localized to the area where the cancer has formed. Obviously, by the time I lost my hair the situation had progressed far beyond what I initially thought, and my brave kids took every new blow in stride.

The night I got home from shaving my head, it was my sweet angel son who came up to me first. Sutton was only eight at the time, and with his precious voice he said, "Mommy, you're beautiful."

If only I could have recorded that interaction and bottled it up forever. I wasn't entirely convinced someone (named John) hadn't told him to say it, but I didn't care. It made all the difference that night and I hold the memory with me now.

Another time we were at a restaurant and he was coloring away, something he doesn't do often. When he finished, he handed his paper to me. It was a beautiful picture of a lion, and on it he'd written, "You're braver than a lion." It was one of the sweetest things that have ever happened to me. Since then, I've surrounded myself with images of lions.

My kids continued to be so incredibly encouraging, considerate, and courageous. I thought for a while that they were putting on a brave face for my benefit, until I realized my kids don't put on a brave face for anything, ever. I once received a photo of Sutton from an apple-picking field trip and it looked like he had been taken hostage. These are not children who can hide their feelings, so thank goodness this was their genuine sentiment.

Neither of them ever asked me to wear a wig or cover my head as my hair slowly started to grow back. I never wanted to put them in the position of having to ask me to wear a head covering, so I kept them carefully in mind every day, to avoid embarrassing them. Somehow, we were all determined to hold each other up and hold ourselves together as a unit. We had never needed to be a team until now.

One Thing

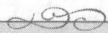

Talking to your kids about a cancer diagnosis and all it could entail (like hair loss) is one of the most difficult pieces of an already very complicated puzzle. It's hard to offer any input or even words of wisdom because it's so personal and unique to each family's circumstances. But here are some nuggets that I observed personally:

1. There will likely be multiple conversations (diagnosis, treatment plan, surgery), so don't feel the need to explain everything all at once. It's not just overwhelming to process, but the initial plan might very well shift as you progress through the journey.

2. As I mentioned previously, talking to your kids in a safe space where they can experience a range of emotions is helpful. They might cry, they might shout, or they might just need to put their head under a pillow. Surrounding them with a comfortable environment helps ease them into the conversation.

3. If your children are old enough to have their own idea of what cancer means, the news will likely come with a lot of understandable fear. But in my experience, the fear starts to fade once they see you are, in fact, doing okay. My kids felt immediate relief once I came home

from the hospital after my double mastectomy and they saw me in one piece.

4. Kids are stronger, braver, and more resilient than they often get credit for. They might ask you very direct questions and are able to handle honest answers. It's quite possible they will surprise you over and over again along the way.

5. Have them make a countdown calendar or do something that involves them in the process. They can cross off every day, circle milestone moments, and celebrate each victory.

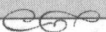

CHAPTER FIFTEEN

Routine, Reclusion, Reflection

For every round of chemo, I was greeted at the cancer center by that comfortable reclining chair with the heat functions. I grew to love that chair. Was it Stockholm syndrome? After that first round when I'd just zoned out, I began to watch television sometimes while the red devil flowed. Usually, I turned on the Food Network. I don't really cook, but watching other people do it was pretty satisfying. And there were always those same two chairs next to me: one for my mom and one for John.

My mom hardly ever missed a chemo appointment. There was one instance, twelve weeks in, when she had to be home for something. But thankfully John was never out of town. He took me to every single doctor's appointment, every round of chemo, all the follow-up appointments, and everything in between. He still does all this, by the way. I know this is not common, and that most people—much less their spouse too—can take only so much time off work. I do not take it for granted for one second.

If you don't have a partner who can help during your treatment period, find a friend or family member who can step up and be that person. Cancer—specifically breast cancer—is so pervasive; this disease hits far and wide. I've become that friend for many, and so many have been that friend for me. If you don't have a friend or family member who can help, there are so many organizations, nonprofits, and even Facebook groups where you can make connections with others who can help.

During my second round of chemo, two weeks after the first round, I surprisingly started to look forward to the routine that followed: a nice lunch followed by a nap. After all, I was now 50 percent done with the red devil, and that was something to celebrate! I still had to wait for the side effects to kick in, but I could officially check off this round on my countdown chart.

That weekend was similar to my first one but more intense. It wasn't the worst thing I'd ever experienced, by any means. It was unpleasant, but it wasn't unbearable. And I know this because my mother took copious notes the entire time. Let's just say I'm known for having a flair for the dramatic, and I think she wanted to fact-check me if I ever claimed it was the worst day of my life.

I saw her thinking that day, *Clea seems fine.* And I genuinely was.

But as I geared up for round three, I started to get nervous. No one gets out of the red devil unscathed, and I knew the rubber was about to hit the road. Physically, at least. I wasn't as prepared for how it would hit mentally.

After ten weeks of cancer treatment—six weeks recovering from my mastectomy and four weeks of chemotherapy—it was taking a toll. Most people in my life had (rightly!) moved on from the frequent check-ins and visits. The cards and flowers had already been sent, the well-wishes wished. I was left missing the normal routines of my life—running errands, dinner with friends, travel for work. It felt like pandemic times, but just for me.

I had this persistent feeling, sort of a pang in my chest. I was getting lonely. Everyone in my household was with me every day, of course, but there was a palpable absence in my life that I couldn't shake. I started to notice that friends who I used to see all the time had disappeared. In sickness and in health doesn't apply to everyone in your life. It felt extra-noticeable compared with some people I hardly ever saw before I was diagnosed (some I hadn't seen in more than a decade) who checked in with John or me pretty regularly during the course of my treatment. Again, cancer is complicated.

Another thing that gave me daily anxiety was how to spend my days. At this point, I wasn't able to work because my mental fatigue and brain fog were as taxing as my physical ailments. I tried to keep up for a while, but it became too difficult and I had to acquiesce. Days seemed to stretch out so far ahead, with no end in sight. Because I'm an extreme extrovert and the opposite of a homebody, this scared me more than most aspects of my condition. Honestly, sitting on a couch all day watching TV sounds like a nightmare to me. But then my mom would make me laugh and say, "Opening cards and receiving packages is a full-time job!" And it was true; though the first wave of cards and flowers had ended, I still received mail now and then (even if most of it was stuff that I had ordered on my own in the middle of the night).

Whether it was an online shopping order or a care package from a friend, the sound of the doorbell made me feel connected to the outside world. It also comprised the majority of my social interaction. Sometimes I would see a delivery person and I wanted to scream out, "Do you want to be friends?" I'm the type of person who goes to a concert and leaves with four phone numbers and lunch plans for the following week with someone I met that night.

But when I think back to some of those deliveries, it wasn't just the human interaction that put a huge smile on my face, it was the fact that someone actually took time out of their life to send something to me. Some of these people I had never even met! John's colleagues, companies that work with The Home Edit, a friend's mom . . . The amount of love I received flowed through my veins and kept me afloat. It brought me to tears more than once.

This is something I always tell people who are sick: Take the wins where you can get them. If it's seeing old friends, getting a boost of energy, or even just having a supportive conversation—store them in a bank. They will continue to provide you with strength and solace.

I received so many special items that I will cherish forever. My friend Haley, who is the world's best gift giver, showed up at my house the night before my surgery with a pair of rainbow (my signature) boxing gloves. She had our various friends write messages of encouragement on them, and when she handed them to me, she told me I needed to remember that I was a fighter. The messages on the glove were written like the ones we would write as kids on the cast of a friend with a broken bone. It was one of the most thoughtful things I have ever received, and the gloves now live on display in our home.

Leah, one of my close friends, is an amazingly talented graphic designer. She made pins and removable tattoos with breast cancer ribbons and the phrase *Clea Kicks Cancer*. She gave them to everyone in my company and our parent company. When I got home from the hospital, the team had put together a compilation video of everyone in the company (and their dogs and kids) wearing the pins and sending me messages.

My joy was beyond words. I had never experienced people being so generous with their time, energy, and effort. I can't quite describe the feeling, but it was something like the world's warmest blanket wrapping around me. People being kind gave me a genuine sense of happiness even when everything else got dark. The stream of love compelled me to keep going.

My friend Merritt, who I've known since birth, made me a curated care package that she knew I would love. She went to one of our favorite shops in New York, Bag-All, and assembled the most special items. She filled a tote bag with a book, a bronze Buddha, and some sweet household things, and she added a gold crossed-fingers pin to the outside of the bag. She also had it embroidered with the phrase *Clea Kicks Cancer*. I took it with me to every single chemo treatment.

You already know I'm an organizer, but I do not hold on to a lot of things. I famously threw out my wedding photos after I had them digitized. John wasn't happy about that one, but the framed pictures were just cluttering up our storage space and had to go. Who needs physical copies? But I *did* keep every single card I received during this period, even the little ones attached to flowers that had been transcribed by the florist. I kept everything I received so I could look at them in their totality and remember how good and kind and loving my friends, family, and even strangers had been in my life.

Knowing that people are thinking about you helps you feel less alone during the hardest times. A little note would honestly change my entire day. It made me feel like each person was right there in the room with me.

This is why when people ask me what they should do for a friend with cancer I say: *Send something—anything.* It doesn't have to be expensive—a handwritten card, a book, a scrap of paper with a flower drawn on it, a treat. Just something that makes them realize they haven't been forgotten. Because there are plenty of days when you feel the world moving on without you, and that silence can be difficult.

People did things for me that they absolutely didn't have to do. Zero people had to get me a single gift, a single floral arrangement, a single basket. Nothing. But they all made such an extraordinary effort to remind me that they cared—which is the reason I kept it all, and why I revisited those gifts again and again over the many months of treatment. They were insulation when the mail dwindled and everything died down.

And the truth was, it was often a struggle to get myself through some of the days that seemingly had no end. It was never a solo fight because I had my loved ones around me, but no one can physically jump into your body and experience what you're feeling at any given moment. That's when I started to lean heavily on my breast cancer friends. We were all in varying degrees of the same situation, and it helped knowing I had people around me who truly understood what I was going through.

We leaned on each other because everyone else in our lives could get only so close to our experience. And everyone else had only so much bandwidth to give. It was an uncomfortable reality when I started to feel a quiet resentment brewing toward everyone who had the luxury of moving on with their lives. It wasn't fair to feel that way, but I felt it nonetheless. I couldn't go five minutes without thinking about cancer, experiencing the side effects of cancer, seeing cancer in the mirror. It's hard to admit, but sometimes I had deep feelings of jealousy. I wanted to be on a summer trip too. I wanted to go to a concert with friends too. I wanted to be able to send a text with a heart and then move on with my day too (although I *did* very much appreciate all the texts with hearts).

That's why having my support group was absolutely critical. We would text all night sometimes, asking each other about new side effects or what a certain chemo round felt like, and comparing how we were feeling. *Has your hair fallen out? Are you feeling nauseous? I started to get joint pain—has that happened to you yet?*

Equally important as having friends experiencing treatment in real time was having a group of survivors to help guide each phase of the process. Being able to talk to women who had already gone through treatment was an absolute lifesaver. Insights about what might happen next and what they had experienced was the only thing I knew I could hold on to. Plus, it kept me off Google. It was so helpful to hear recommendations for how to deal with certain ailments, tips for what types of lotion helped soothe scars, how to ice my port, you name it.

Information helped ease my mind because being prepared is my love language. I truly felt if I just bought the right cooling pillow, my life would get exponentially easier to manage. So I continued to compile lists of suggestions and try out different items and techniques. Having an action item meant I was doing something to control the situation as best I could. Control the controllables. And it turned out I needed all the prep I could get before diving into round three.

One Thing

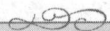

Loneliness is a very common feeling when you have cancer, even when you're surrounded by loved ones. Don't be concerned or ashamed if it creeps in every so often. When I was experiencing bouts of loneliness, I found the best remedy was some form of escapism. I needed to focus on someone else's life for a little while and have other characters be my company.

Some people might choose reality TV, but for me, it was always a book on my Kindle. When I was going through my cancer battle, I read forty-eight books. As soon as one ended, I started a new one in my queue. Books became my constant companions, and the habit didn't stop after I rang the bell. They are still my respite, because to this day, I sometimes experience the same feelings. The emotional ups and downs of cancer linger, and it's helpful to find something you can always turn to.

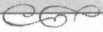

CHAPTER SIXTEEN

The Last Round

I had gotten through the first two rounds of chemo relatively unscathed, but after the third round I felt much worse. Of course, I anticipated this would be the case, but it was unnerving to experience such unpredictability.

The worst thing by far I experienced after round three was heartburn. Admittedly, I had never had heartburn before and always thought it was no big deal. I mean, if a bottle of Tums could handle it, how bad could it be? Well, it turns out it could be *very* bad. I would wake up at night, every hour, choking on whatever bile was coming up. After everything I had already been through, I refused to accept that heartburn was taking me down. But sure enough, it was. I couldn't sleep, I couldn't work—it became completely debilitating.

No over-the-counter remedies were even remotely working, so I called Dr. Kurtz to help find a solution. She ended up calling in a medication laced with lidocaine that would literally numb my throat. *Wow*, was it gross. Ironic that the thing that was supposed to stop me from gagging was making me gag.

I went back to my friends who had already been through the red devil to piece together what I had left to expect. Everyone gave me similar feedback: I was going to feel like absolute shit, and then it was going to be over. Noted.

"Okay, but can you explain the *level* of shit that I'm going to feel like?" I asked. "How bad will it be?"

I knew that no one could predict how I was going to feel, but even the smallest insight helped me feel like I was in control. Knowing what was coming made me feel more prepared and less worried. It's kind of like when the pilot comes on the overhead speaker saying there's turbulence ahead. You can't actually *do* anything about it, but at least you expect it when it happens. It's one thing to feel something physically intense, but it's another to be surprised by it.

One of the reasons I am writing this book is to give other people with cancer the same comfort I felt when I was talking to my network. To inform them what might happen at each stage so they are not so caught off guard. I know that everyone experiences each type of cancer differently, but there's enough common ground and shared experience to unite everyone battling this disease. Talking with people who have been through or are going through something similar is invaluable.

By the time I got to the fourth round, I was extremely nervous. The first two rounds weren't so bad, but the third was *rough*, with that terrible heartburn along with all the nausea, bone pain, muscle aches, and fatigue. What on earth was the fourth going to feel like? I wasn't surprised when it started off just like the others. The nurses greeted us with big smiles and made their rounds, bringing snacks and warm blankets. They could honestly make time spent in the chemo chair feel outright pleasant. Between that and getting my little lunch and nap afterward, I could almost forget the reality of what was happening.

One thing that didn't sink in for a while was just how toxic chemo drugs are (which sounds obvious, but there were a lot of things to process, and this simply wasn't one of them). There is a photo John took during the third round, in which one of the nurses is administering the initial drug wearing a full biohazard suit with a mask, head covering, and gloves. Until I saw the photo, it hadn't occurred to me that she needed to suit up to just be holding the drug, while I was literally getting it pumped into my veins. It was an eye-opening experience to realize I was marching day by day through this, checking off boxes, but maybe not fully wrapping my head around the extent of what I was experiencing.

The day after my fourth round was administered, I started to feel the effects. Usually, I didn't feel too bad until the Saturday after. But this time, I started to feel sick within twenty-four hours. By the time Saturday came around, I was the sickest I have ever felt in my life. I spent the entire day in my medical recliner at home, floating in and out of consciousness. My whole body hurt. Even my skin was sensitive to the touch. I was so nauseated, but I had to eat to take my medication; I was so tired, but I wasn't comfortable enough to sleep; I wanted to distract myself, but my eyes were too blurry to focus on a book or the TV. I was just encased in a dense fog I couldn't see my way out of. All I could do was ride it out and hope it would be over soon.

At one point, I remember thinking to myself in between the drifting, *Am I dying? And if I'm not dying, then what could dying possibly feel like?*

I felt like I was almost levitating over myself. I kept picturing the nurse administering the drugs that were so clearly dangerous to be exposed to, which were now coursing through my body. What if they had crossed the line from helping to hurting? No. I was going to push that thought far away and not panic. To be honest, I was too weak to panic anyway, so at least my brain and my body agreed about that.

The only good memory I have about that day (I'm grateful to have even one) is that my mother and I decided on a TV marathon to kill time. Through months of surgery and chemo I had yet to turn on the TV during the day until that point—all the TV watching I'd done had been at night. I think I had memories of watching TV during the day as a child home sick from school, and I didn't want to perpetually feel like a kid with the flu.

I landed on season eleven of *Top Chef*. The stakes were just high enough to hold my interest, but low enough that I could doze off occasionally and it wouldn't matter. My mother and I watched the entire thing, all fourteen hours. I didn't have the energy to laugh at the time, but while we were watching, I realized that my mother had never watched a competition show before. She barely watches TV in general, and certainly not fourteen hours of cooking challenges. So, as I was sitting there, drifting in and out of sleep, my mother was pacing back and forth in the living room, so stressed that someone she liked was being sent home.

"He was *robbed*! And he has a newborn baby!" she screamed at the TV about one of the contestants, and then she delivered an oration worthy of Model UN about another's worthiness for the finale.

She was *so invested*. It's become a joke between us now that when my mom comes to spend time with me after surgeries, we sense another round of *Top Chef* in our future. At least now I hope she's braced herself for the ups and downs of reality TV.

I did end up making it through that Saturday somehow. I don't remember eating. I don't even remember sleeping. I was in an absolute haze for twenty-four hours. But when I woke up on Sunday, I felt significantly improved. I didn't feel well, but I felt better. I was elated as I walked into the kitchen to deliver the good news.

In that moment, I remember thinking that I was over the mountain. Nothing was going to be worse than the red devil, and I had just gotten through the hardest recovery day. Taxol was supposed to be a much easier experience, and subsequent radiation was supposed to be even easier. So in my mind, that Sunday equaled a huge victory. With a big smile on my face, I started planning *two* celebratory trips: one to Hawaii (my happy place) with the family at the end of treatment, and then one to Italy (I had never been) the following May with just John. For the first time since I'd been diagnosed with cancer, I had a new lease on life.

I took my win and kept marching toward the finish line. I had a couple of weeks off between my final round of AC and my first round of Taxol, so John and I also planned a brief summer trip to Los Angeles. It felt like a great time to visit family and have a little fun for the first time in months.

One Thing

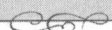

I realize planning two big celebratory trips (three if you count Los Angeles) is quite extravagant. Looking back, I'm not sure we needed to fly over so many oceans. But I felt like I had to shock my system with excitement to see the light at the end of the tunnel. And it really did help to have those trips to look forward to.

Think of a place that brings you comfort—a lake house, the beach, or anywhere that makes you happy—and promise yourself you will get there as soon as you're able. During the long weeks and months of cancer treatment, I would spend time visualizing being away, researching things to do or restaurants to try. If I couldn't sleep, I would picture myself relaxing by the water reading a book and it would calm me down. Of course, it's always nice to have something to look forward to, but when you have cancer it's even more of a gift because it also helps you visualize life beyond being sick all the time.

CHAPTER SEVENTEEN

It's Not Over, Is It?

As our L.A. vacation approached, I found myself getting *very* excited for what had always been a routine trip to see family. I was going to cherish every single place I went for the rest of my life. Being confined to the house for so many months made me long to be on an airplane, and I don't even like to fly. I started to spend my downtime daydreaming about places I would go once I had the opportunity. If literally any future work trip was being considered, my answer was going to be yes, no questions asked. I finally allowed myself to consider what life would be like after treatment was behind me. I hadn't given in to that temptation before because I needed to focus on the present in order to pull my way through each day. But now I was allowing the light to break through.

Even before I got sick, I didn't ever give myself downtime. I was always working and was moving nonstop. And I don't say that in a negative way—I thrived in that type of environment. I loved every minute of my fast-paced life. I truly couldn't remember the last time I had just completely taken time off to do nothing. Cancer, for better or worse, was pushing me to do just that. Which is why

I keep repeating that cancer is complicated. With all the hard and painful moments, there are extremely cherished ones at the same time. The world around you comes more into focus. You take less for granted. You want to live every minute of your life in a way you'll remember.

So even going on a very mundane trip to California made me absolutely ecstatic. I had to get clearance from my doctors in order to get on an airplane because my immune system was so compromised, but because I had waited a couple of weeks after my last chemo round, my white blood cell count had rebounded enough to allow me to travel.

When we arrived at the hotel in Los Angeles, I nearly cried from happiness. A *hotel*! It had been so long! I was so happy for a change of scenery, room service, and a fluffy bathrobe. During the day, John and I would sit by the pool while the kids swam, and we'd host various friends and family as they came to say hi or eat lunch. It was so nice to sit in the sunshine and get a few moments of pure enjoyment.

In an effort to make things as fun as possible for the kids, we decided to go to Disneyland for the day with our friends. Should I have gone to Disneyland in the middle of chemo? Probably not! But I figured if I rented a scooter to drive around the park, I would be able to manage. It was the summer, so it was quite hot that day, but I kept as hydrated as possible, and I only walked as I was getting on and off rides. Still, I noticed that my movements felt labored. I soon became *exhausted*. I found myself anxiously wanting to leave and get in bed—which had pretty much never happened to me.

The next day we took it easy and hung out by the pool again. I had a couple of friends over to the hotel restaurant for lunch, but beyond that, we were mostly lounging. The only times I had to get up were to use the restroom. Which wasn't that far . . . so why was I so out of breath? Surely walking the length of the pool shouldn't have been enough to elevate my heart rate. So why was it beating out of my chest? It wasn't normal. But nothing is normal during chemo. There was such a laundry list of side effects that I guessed what I was experiencing was one of them. I figured my body was just exhausted from fighting the war.

Still, I wondered if maybe I should call the doctor, just to ask if this was typical. There were so many things constantly popping up—heartburn, nausea, fatigue, joint pain, body aches—maybe this was just going to be added to the list. It couldn't hurt to check.

I reached out to my oncologist and my primary care doctor thinking they would give me a quick reply confirming that what I was feeling was normal. They both said the one thing you never want a doctor to say: "That's unusual."

What? Nothing is "unusual" during chemo. Every single, solitary thing you can imagine is possible. Except for this, apparently. It was decided that I should head to the emergency room at Cedars-Sinai in Los Angeles and get checked out.

The last thing I wanted to do was visit an ER. It was the last thing my doctors wanted too, because I was so susceptible to infection. Was it worse to let these symptoms stretch on, or was it worse to risk being around infectious germs? Ultimately, I accepted that I had to go, but I prayed it wouldn't take long.

I only needed a few tests. The primary concern seemed to be potential blood clots in my legs, which can occur during treatment. Again, you're kind of at risk for everything, which is why I couldn't believe the symptoms I was experiencing were cause for concern. But it was critical to rule out the blood clots because if I had them it would mean I couldn't fly home.

We had flown our family assistant to L.A. with us for extra help, so thankfully she was able to watch the kids while John and I headed to the emergency room. Everyone was calm, except for me; I was dreading the experience. The only time I had ever been in the emergency room—and ironically it was this exact emergency room at Cedars—was when I was in labor. *Verrrrry* different experience.

The ER was horrifying. It was actually worse than I had expected. There were people sleeping on the floor inside and on the ground outside. There were people fighting, screaming, begging, coughing, bleeding, you name it. There were people in wheelchairs, in makeshift hospital beds, in a COVID tent, and some being led out by police in handcuffs. It was so crowded that in the end I opted to stand outside because my immune system was compromised.

Once we had checked in, a nurse came outside to introduce herself; she had been made aware of my circumstances through Vanderbilt. She said she would give us updates, but that they were backed up and obviously overcrowded. Every couple of hours, I was called back to do something like get my blood pressure and vitals taken, but then I was sent back outside to wait. I would come in to get blood drawn, and then go back outside to wait. It went on like this for about six hours. It was getting cold, but I was too afraid to go inside.

Finally, a room opened up and we were escorted down the hallway. The situation in the waiting room was nothing compared with the hospital itself. There were people screaming from bed restraints and threatening us as we walked by, people being treated in hallway hospital beds only covered by umbrellas. It felt apocalyptic.

Even in our room, I could hear screams of pain and shouts of profanity from down the hall. For the 758th time that day, I considered making a run for it. Except I was at the hospital because I was having trouble literally walking around, let alone running anywhere. I had no choice but to shake it off, put on my hospital gown, and wait for the doctor.

By that point I had been there for eight hours and was so hungry I was about to eat the hospital bed. One of the nurses managed to find me some peanut butter crackers and a little water bottle, and it felt like I had just eaten a three-course meal from my favorite restaurant. As another hour passed, I continued to check in with my doctors in Nashville to give them updates. The ER doctor on call finally visited my room to tell me about all the tests I'd be receiving and inform me that he would like me to stay overnight. My oncologist and my primary care doctor were split on what I should do at this point: Should I stay in the emergency room, or was I diminishing my returns at this point? We decided to split the difference and stay for the results but not spend the night.

I ended up at the hospital until four a.m., with good news and bad news. The good news was that I was clear for blood clots—that was a huge deal because it meant I could travel back to Nashville. The bad news was that my blood panel showed that my red blood cell count was basically down to nothing, which explained why I was so weak and short of breath. The doctor explained that I needed an emergency blood transfusion, and that he didn't want me to leave the hospital without getting one. I was desperate to get out of there and back to the hotel. I was still in touch with my doctors in Nashville (bless them), and they gave me the green light to get the transfusion back at home. I just had to *get* home as soon as possible.

Because I couldn't risk infection and needed to leave the next day, we had to charter a small plane to get us back to Nashville. It was an emergency, but I was so mad at myself for putting us in this situation. I could have avoided all this, and the huge cost of flying private, but I was trying to have a normal and carefree vacation, when nothing about my present life was normal and carefree. I had no business traipsing around Los Angeles and scootering around Disneyland. I needed to keep prioritizing my health even when I didn't feel like it. There would be plenty of fun times ahead, but I needed to stop flying so close to the sun.

One Thing

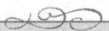

While cancer is an equal-opportunity illness and doesn't discriminate between who it affects, the medical treatment a person receives can really vary based on many factors, including socioeconomic status, race, gender, and geographical location. In this case, I was lucky enough to be able to fly back to Nashville for treatment instead of staying in Los Angeles, but for many, there are few options available. Thankfully, there are a host of excellent organizations that can provide cancer patients with advocacy, financial assistance, housing, and overall support. Research both national and local organizations, but here are a few standout groups that can offer help:

- American Cancer Society
- Stand Up to Cancer
- St. Jude
- Good Days
- American Cancer Fund

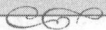

One More Thing

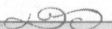

It's often hard to know when you might be overdoing things until it's too late. But if you listen to your body, you can likely catch something abnormal before you land yourself in the hospital. I clearly did *not* listen or act quickly, and I paid the price for it. When you are undergoing cancer treatment, you can experience a sort of medical fatigue. You are constantly being poked and prodded and tested, and having to go to even one more doctor appointment feels like a bridge too far. Or maybe it even feels unnecessary because surely whatever is bothering you would have been caught at one of the other million appointments. But it's so important to keep a watchful eye on the way you are feeling day in and day out. Whether it's via a mental check-in, talking to your friends and saying it out loud, or writing it down in a journal, it will help you stay accountable for what you're experiencing.

Even with medical fatigue, remember to check in with your doctor if you're starting to feel something that just doesn't seem normal. I waited way too long to ask my doctor if my shortness of breath and rapid heart rate were problematic. All it took was one quick conversation before I was sent to the ER because what I was experiencing was *not* normal. Sometimes you must push yourself into vigilance even when you're exhausted, don't feel like it, or worried you're overreacting. You will never regret reaching out for answers, but you might very well regret staying silent.

CHAPTER EIGHTEEN

Up All Night

I received my blood transfusion as soon as I got back to Nashville, and I immediately felt better. It's wild that I allowed myself to feel so poorly for so long without asking questions. Had I learned nothing? If you feel something, say something! There's no prize for suffering in silence.

Now that my red blood cell count was back up, I could start the next phase of chemo: twelve rounds of Taxol across twelve weeks. Almost everyone agrees that Taxol is a much easier experience than AC, so I wasn't terribly nervous given what I had already been through. I had convinced myself it was going to be a comparative walk in the park. Which *basically* meant I was practically finished and totally done! You've heard of "girl math"? (If it's on sale, somehow you've actually made money buying it.) Try the even more reality-denying "girl-with-cancer math." Even with five months left of treatment (twelve rounds of Taxol across twelve weeks and then six weeks of radiation five days a week), I considered myself practically over the finish line.

Taxol is easier to tolerate than AC, but the downside is that it's also administered once a week. Not only do you lose the extra week to recover physically but you also don't have that extra time to recover mentally. Receiving chemo every week, in a continual cycle, takes a toll on your mind and body even if you feel less sick. All that said, I felt pretty confident that I could crush the remainder of chemo. Let's go, Taxol.

The infusion itself was a very different process from AC because Taxol has the potential to cause an allergic reaction as soon as it's administered. Beforehand, you're given pre-meds like Benadryl and, most significantly, a hefty dose of steroids to help prevent a reaction. My nurse (who had been with me during my AC days too) actually had to stay in the room with me as I started receiving the drug in case she had to immediately shut the chemo pump off. Was this comforting or terrifying?

I tried to remain calm and just assume I would be fine. But I did get nervous as all this was happening. For the first time, I had anxiety about *receiving* chemo, rather than just the side effects from it. Until then, I had mostly been focused on not throwing up after the fact; I hadn't even considered that I could have a reaction in the moment.

Another very weird part about Taxol infusions compared with AC is that it's recommended you ice your hands and feet the whole time. The drug can cause neuropathy in your extremities (numbness or weakness that usually shows up in hands and feet), and the ice helps prevent that from happening. The red devil was awful for a million reasons, but at least being freezing cold was not one of them. Still, I was committed to getting through this Taxol experience relatively unscathed, so I diligently wore my ice mitts and ice booties.

Chemo comes with a lot of rules and recommendations, so ice

mitts were just another addition to the list. Chemo rules are not dissimilar to pregnancy rules. There were foods I couldn't eat, like raw vegetables and sushi, because I needed to avoid a bacterial infection at all costs. I have to admit, at first I didn't take it as seriously as I should have. I mean, I had *cancer.* I doubted crudités and dip were going to send me to the grave. But my nurse finally told me point-blank that a carrot stick quite literally *could* kill me, and that I had to act accordingly.

Well, that did the trick! No more salads and spicy tuna rolls. My doctor reminded me that bacterial infections were even more serious than COVID because my compromised immune system had a better chance fighting viruses than bacteria.

With all these risk calculations in my head, I didn't even think to question the amount of steroids I was receiving. They were a necessary piece of this puzzle, so I accepted whatever was being administered. I never even remotely considered that they would become one of the hardest parts of my treatment. I was used to the usual wave of Thursday infusions, Friday feeling iffy, Saturday feeling sick, and Sunday starting to rebound. What I didn't anticipate is that in addition to this cycle, I could not sleep *at all.* Without exaggeration, the steroids kept me awake every hour of every single night. It was, in a word, hell.

I was desperate to get some rest. Not sleeping was a different kind of torture than any of the sickness I'd experienced thus far. With every day that passed, I felt myself mentally reaching a breaking point.

By July, in my third week on Taxol, and my third week of no sleep, we headed just outside Nashville because our nanny at the time was getting married. It was a beautiful outdoor summer wedding, which meant it was as hot as it was lovely. I was wearing a full-length dress, and a wig with long hair. I was exhausted from not sleeping and overheated from the humidity, and I kept needing to sit down because it was hard to be on my feet. While everyone was enjoying cocktail hour, I had to sit in the church with my family for some much-needed air-conditioning. Once the reception began, I couldn't eat the meal because I was so nauseated—but not eating also nauseated me, so I nibbled on bread. I was so frustrated. I was angry and tired and felt like life had become unfair. The old "why me" feelings were creeping back, and they were hard to fight off.

When we got home that night, I took my wig off as fast as I could and went out on the back porch to sit in my chair. Well, it had *become* my chair. It was where I had been spending all my time since my surgery and subsequent treatment began in April. It was where I would read my book or listen to music, or sit and chat with my mom while waiting for the kids to get home from school. And I would sit there in the middle of the night when I couldn't sleep . . . which was now every night at all hours.

That chair on the screened-in porch was my source of comfort and solace. It was therapeutic. For some of my cancer friends, that was a bench in Central Park or a spot on the beach. For me, it was my chair on the porch, especially on summer nights, when I could take my wig off and sit peacefully in the warm air.

But this night, after the wedding, it was anything but peaceful. I started sobbing—shoulders shaking, hunched over, and wailing. I was just *so* sick of being sick. I hadn't slept in weeks and I felt like I couldn't keep going. Any end in sight I had previously glimpsed had vanished, and I couldn't tell up from down as the waves of hopelessness crashed around me.

My mom wasn't in town that particular week, and I realized in that moment I needed her desperately. I cried and screamed, "I miss my mom! I want my *mom!*" My kids came out to the porch to comfort me, and I was too wrapped up in despair to put on a brave face. They somehow weren't afraid of my reaction; it's like they understood it. I was sick and wanted my mom to be with me. Nothing is more universal than that sentiment.

I had been strong through so much, and that night the floodgates just opened. I felt sorry for myself, which is a feeling I can't stand. I'd allow it briefly, but then I had to get to work on a solution. I'm nothing if not goal-oriented, and I was going to get through this. It took all my determination to say, "Clea, you need to remember the lesson you learned at the beginning of this journey. You need to speak up, advocate for yourself, talk to the doctors, and tell them something is wrong."

I was tired of being miserable. I think as cancer patients we forget that we don't necessarily have to live that way.

First thing in the morning, I called Dr. Park. "I can't sleep for more than an hour at a time, and nothing seems to work," I said. "I genuinely feel like I am losing it, like I'm going crazy."

Why was I still so stubborn about not speaking up as soon as something was wrong? Every time I did, my doctors listened to me and immediately worked out a solution. My oncologist suggested lowering my steroid dose for the upcoming week—round four—because I hadn't had any allergic reaction to date. My sleep medication was also increased to include Ativan *plus* Benadryl to cut through the effects from the steroids. I believe that combo was referred to as an "elephant dart." Which, to be honest, I needed.

"We have to get you sleeping," Dr. Kurtz said. "If you don't get sleep, your body won't be able to handle anything else."

The next week, I showed up to my chemo appointment and sat down for my vitals and blood panel as I always did. It's crucial to make sure that your white blood cell count is high enough that you can receive chemotherapy. If it's not, they send you home and delay your treatment. I had been sent home once during round two, and I didn't want it to happen again. Unfortunately, my white blood cell count was too low for me to receive chemotherapy that week.

Clearly, my white blood cells were struggling to keep up with the one-week recovery schedule. The brief time between treatments wasn't enough to rehabilitate my white blood cell count, so we started using growth factor support shots—a bone marrow stimulant used to push your body to produce white blood cells. During AC, these shots are a given because you are so severely depleted that you need it, but usually patients are able to rebound on Taxol. Still, I figured it wasn't a big deal to go back to that option because it had worked well in the past—what could be the downside? The nurses would just tape the delivery mechanism to my arm like a diabetes glucose meter, and then twenty-four hours later, it would start ticking like a time bomb before it injected into my arm. It didn't hurt, it was just jarring. Like a wound-up jack-in-the-box you know is about to spring out at you. But it works!

The bad news about delaying treatment by another week is that it also delayed my completion date. But the good news for me was that it meant a week with no steroids. Maybe with my new medication routine I would actually be able to sleep!

It took a few days, but for the first time in a long time, I got four hours of sleep in a row instead of one. I was still up in the middle of the night, in my chair on the back porch, but I felt like I had gained a little bit of control back.

One Thing

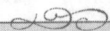

For me, moving from AC to Taxol was a good reminder that one treatment isn't better or worse, or easier versus harder. They are both distinct and have challenges that vary from week to week and case by case. I declared victory after my fourth round of AC, assuming everything else was going to be a breeze in comparison—but Taxol knocked me down to the ground in a very different and draining way. It turns out (shockingly!) there is no *better* or *easier* when it comes to cancer, only unexpected twists and turns and ups and downs.

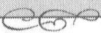

CHAPTER NINETEEN

Ringing the Bell

I was finally ready to get my fourth round of Taxol. The supplemental shots had worked, and I was back on track. I had lost two weeks due to the white blood cell count delays, but that wasn't too bad. And this time, my steroids would be lowered significantly, so I was less fearful of the sleepless nights to follow. I was managing my other side effects pretty well, and I was ready to celebrate being 33 percent finished with Taxol. In just eight more weeks, I would be on the other side.

As round five approached, I crossed my fingers. I sat in the chemo chair piled up with blankets and snacks awaiting the go-ahead from my nurse. But when she walked into my room, I knew from her facial expression that my numbers still weren't high enough to receive treatment. It was time to pack up because chemo wasn't going to be happening. It's one thing to have an occasional reprieve, but I was never going to get through this if I wasn't receiving treatment. The eight weeks I had accounted for in my head just ticked over to nine weeks instead. Like last time, I received my growth support shot and headed home. And like last time, the following week my count improved and I was able to get round five.

By the time I walked in for round six, I didn't get too comfortable—which was good because my numbers had plummeted again. This was getting very frustrating. At this point, I was a full month behind where I thought I would be. It's hard to imagine *wanting* to get chemo, but not getting it was just delaying the inevitable. The growth support shot went into my arm, and I received round six the following week.

I sat down for round seven already expecting the worst. But this time, when my nurse walked into the room she said to expect a call from my doctor. Right then, my phone started ringing.

"Clea," Dr. Park said, "I think we have to call it. I think you're done."

I said, "I'm sorry, *what?*"

"You've received a lot of chemotherapy already. You did four rounds of AC and six rounds of Taxol. The twelve rounds of Taxol is the standard of care, but there is no evidence to suggest exactly twelve rounds is what an individual needs to receive. Right now, if we keep going, there's a possibility it will do more harm than good. Your body might stop being able to produce *any* blood cells at all." He underscored what I already knew, which is everyone responds to treatment differently. "I think your body is just done. I think it's time we stop." He asked, "How do you feel about stopping now?"

"Are you *kidding me?!* *I get to stop?* I'm actually done?" I couldn't get out of that treatment chair fast enough. I almost yelled into the phone, "No backsies!" I was going to get out of there before anyone changed their mind.

I looked up at John as I ended the call. I could tell we were both thinking the same thing: *This is the moment we've been waiting for.* It was finally going to be over.

"How do you feel about it?" he asked me.

We both knew that there was more of a safety net from receiving twelve rounds instead of only six. But we also needed to remember that I had to listen to my body, and my body was telling me it was done. And in a rare moment of alignment, my brain agreed.

Largely, I think I was just in disbelief. I had gone into the breast center that morning thinking it was time for another round, and that hopefully I would have five rounds left. I never expected that it would actually be *over*. My mother wasn't even in town to witness it! As I got up from the chair and walked out of the room, the entire nursing staff was clapping and cheering. They had even made a banner and signed a certificate that I had completed chemotherapy. Then I got to do the very big, very exciting thing I had been looking forward to: I got to ring the bell.

I couldn't believe it. I hadn't prepared for this moment at all. I honestly would've worn something better had I known there would be photos. Maybe put on some makeup. But no, instead I was in my pajamas and as bald as can be. But I was smiling from ear to ear and jumping up and down. This moment was nothing short of pure elation.

The only thing missing was that my mother wasn't there with me. She had spent so many hours sitting in her chair next to mine, and she didn't get to have the big payoff. I called her the second I walked outside to tell her the good news, and of course she was thrilled. Although she asked me 67,854,763 times if I was *sure* I didn't need to continue. I imagined her calling Dr. Park on the side to confirm my story. She knew all the nurses by name, so she could certainly collect a full report.

Throughout this part of my journey, there were so many surreal moments, so many excruciating moments, so many scary moments. But I say *cancer is complicated* so often because there were also so many loving moments, special moments, moments of togetherness that I will hold with me forever. I will truly never watch *Top Chef* the same way again.

I was grateful for the ups to counteract the downs. Had you asked me at the start of my diagnosis if I anticipated any good moments in addition to the bad, I would have thought the question insane.

One of my biggest fears following my diagnosis was how my quality of life would be affected. I was so worried that every day would feel like a giant rain cloud was following me around. So, you can imagine my surprise when I realized I was still laughing, still able to go places, still able to enjoy moments with friends and family. I would have saved myself a lot of additional stress if I had believed this would be possible.

I also learned that the cancer roller coaster is ongoing, both physically and mentally. Starting from the day of my first surgery, everything could and did change in the blink of an eye. I was learning how to be comfortable with being uncomfortable. Not the easiest thing to manage when you're a control freak.

Before cancer, I truly thought I was a delicate flower. But I was able to handle so much more—*so* much more—than I ever thought possible. And some of those times you fight like hell, and some of those times, you learn when to call it. If you're laboring while you're walking, if you're feeling terrible, if your heart is beating out of your chest, if you're not able to sleep, or if your white blood cell count refuses to rebound—then your body is telling you something. And it's begging you to actually listen.

One Thing

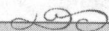

Think positive thoughts. I know it sounds like a cliché, but bear with me. Looking for the positive moments helps disrupt the inevitable barrage of negativity that comes with cancer. One of the reasons why I wanted to name this book *Cancer Is Complicated* is because this disease provides nuance. It is possible to feel terrified while also feeling great comfort. As patients, we deal with the circumstances handed to us, we deal with the deep love we receive, we deal with the crushing fear we experience. All can be true at the same time.

Positive thinking was not something I normally practiced; I've always been more of the anxious-worrier type. But if you want to keep your head above water during cancer, you need to grasp every positive moment and thought that you can. It might be someone stopping by, a card you get in the mail, your kids saying something funny, a flower that blooms in your backyard, or a million and one other things. Do your best to collect each one.

Here are some ideas for how to practice noticing and collecting these moments:

- **Write them down in a journal.** If you are a pen-to-paper type of person, a daily journal is a great method to capture these moments.

- **Record them in the Notes app.** Personally, I'm not a paper person and always opt for digital note-taking.

- **Social media.** I also decided to document positive moments online. Not just so I could look back and remember how I felt on a given day, but so other people could follow along during their journey as well.

- **Mental notes.** You don't have to write anything down if you prefer to hold on to your own thoughts. Simply taking some time at the end of the day to reflect on something good that happened does wonders.

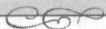

CHAPTER TWENTY

The Rundown on Radiation

Since the beginning of treatment, the plan had been the same: Recover from my double mastectomy, complete chemo, and complete radiation. Now that I had completed AC, aka the red devil, and Taxol, it was time for radiation.

I have to admit, before my diagnosis I didn't quite know the difference between chemo and radiation. All I knew was that chemo had a reputation for being absolutely horrific, but there were no main characters in movies getting sick from radiation.

The difference was ultimately explained to me like this: Both therapies kill cancer cells, but in different ways. Chemotherapy drugs are designed to kill and shrink cancer cells throughout the entire body. Radiation treatment is localized to the area where the tumor or tumors first formed. This is my not-scientific-or-in-any-way-exact description of what I gathered at the beginning of this process.

There are situations different from mine, as when a tumor is isolated without spreading elsewhere and only surgery is needed. Early on, that's what I'd hoped for, that the tumors were localized in my right breast and had not entered my lymph nodes. I've had plenty of friends who were able to opt for a lumpectomy; everyone experiences a different path. And let me just say for the record that I have no patience for who-had-it-worse competitions. Cancer is cancer. However many rounds of chemo and radiation someone receives, or if they receive no rounds at all; whether you receive one surgery or ten; whether someone is a survivor or previvor (meaning they have surgery in hopes of avoiding future complications)—this is a world no one asked to be in, and everyone deserves the same respect.

It's pretty clear that I'm not a doctor, but it's worth repeating, and I will say this a hundred times: I am not giving medical advice for what you should or should not do, or what you need or don't need. But it's well known that not everyone who has cancer must receive chemo and/or radiation. Again, I was told it was *possible* that I wasn't going to need chemo because my initial biopsy had showed that my tumors were confined to my right breast. But of course, during surgery, when they found the cancer had in fact spread to my lymph nodes, the trajectory of my life changed considerably.

Because my cancer journey was very public and I had a social media following, people were reaching out to me, weighing in, and sending messages all the time. Some of those people were friends, but most were strangers. What I started to realize through my messages was that no one mentioned radiation being a breeze. I had hoped for some "This will be nothing compared to chemo!" DMs. But the majority were variations of a sad face emoji and good luck wishes.

Some people would even share horror stories with me about the severity of burns that radiation caused. They wanted to caution me or recommend a certain cream due to my very fair skin. I couldn't even walk around on a sunny day without SPF, and now I was going to be radiated—how was that going to work? I didn't have an answer, but I diligently bought all the creams they suggested (I used an ultrarich face cream instead of a typical body cream because it's extra delicate and made for sensitive skin) and took all their notes seriously.

I also knew that my radiation experience might even be worse than some other breast cancer patients' because they had to treat my right armpit in addition to my breast. The entire offending area was going to be zapped, which was a little nerve-racking. The thought of my skin burning—or worse, tearing—in my armpit seemed extra painful.

To add insult to injury, the beam wasn't going to be able to effectively target my right side due to my left breast expander being in the way—which meant the left breast had to be deflated to avoid any issues. If they didn't, there could be a host of potential problems with the beam hitting areas like the heart or lungs. The last thing you want is your radiologist winging it. So even though I knew the reasoning behind the decision, it was still pretty mortifying walking around with my left breast much flatter than my right. In clothing, I could fake it with inserts, but it was uncomfortable for me to look in a mirror. Still, if deflating the little volleyball I had in my chest was going to be the solution, I was happy to do it.

Thinking about it now, there is so much about cancer treatment that seems to be weirdly simple, almost primitive. It was the same thought I had every time I went into surgery and had the doctors initialing and drawing on me with a Sharpie. Modern medicine has come so far, and yet there are certain things that have never really evolved. In some ways, maybe that can be reassuring. When certain solutions are more low tech, they can seem more tangible and easy to understand. I can't read a printout report on my breast, but I sure can recognize a Sharpie mark.

Reminding myself of this helped keep me levelheaded as I prepared for my first radiation treatment. Between all the good luck messages, the horror stories, and the 5 percent of people who weren't fazed by it at all, I'd heard a lot about what I might experience. I had a couple of weeks between my last chemo infusion and my first radiation appointment, so I pondered the different outcomes incessantly. While I had endless information, so much was still unknowable. The truth was, I wouldn't have all the answers until I went into the treatment room myself.

One Thing

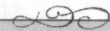

My Radiation Must-Haves:

- Extra-rich cream (Eucerin Advanced Repair is a really good one and available everywhere)

- Miaderm lotion (helps to soothe irritation from the burn)

- Aquaphor for any flaky skin or areas that itch

- Loose-fitting cotton tops

- Bras without underwire (or no bra at all most days!)

- A cooling pillow

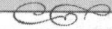

CHAPTER TWENTY-ONE

My First Treatment

A s I walked around with my left side deflated, I was grateful when I found out my radiation schedule had been moved up thanks to my chemo sessions ending early. But being moved up in the calendar also meant I was starting sooner than expected—once again thwarting my meticulous planning. When it was time for my first radiation treatment at the beginning of October, I was pretty nervous. But that didn't stop me from feeling grateful that I was able to start the next step.

Radiation, from when you walk into the room to when you leave it, is pretty quick. It's *much* faster than chemotherapy. You can literally do it on your lunch break and then go back to work. The radiation plan that was suggested for me was for six weeks, five days a week—a total of thirty rounds. That's something a lot of people don't mention, and it's important to wrap your head around. Five days a week is not easy to prepare for. So even though radiation is much faster than chemotherapy, it's on your mind all the time because it occurs almost every single day and you have to schedule your life around it.

For the thirty rounds of radiation, I decided to keep a mental countdown of all of my sessions. I had done it throughout AC, counting down from four. I'd had a countdown started for Taxol too, and I finished ahead of schedule, ending at six. And now it was time to start the clock over for radiation. It was helpful to have an end in sight. I would start off with thirty sessions and then cross off every single one, until I was able to ring the bell for the last time. That gave me some benchmarks, which helped with my motivation and determination. When I went to the first appointment, I thought to myself, *Okay, look at that. I'm no longer at thirty. Now I'm going to be at twenty-nine.*

Walking into the massive building where I was going to receive radiation was already a different experience than entering the Vanderbilt-Ingram Cancer Center, where I'd received my infusions. Vanderbilt was blessedly in my neighborhood, whereas this building was part of the medical main campus in midtown. Main campus is where I went for all my surgeries, and where I would now go for radiation. I had to take the elevator down to the basement. Precautions are taken to shield other people from the radiation that patients receive. It was kind of a maze down there, and with each turn, my anxiety increased—probably due in part to the fact that I knew that without help I'd never be able to find the elevator again.

When John and I finally reached the waiting room, I checked in on the computer and waited to be called in. Even after hearing so many radiation reports, I wondered what it would feel like to receive this kind of treatment myself for the first time. I finally heard my name called, received a good luck kiss from John, and was escorted to a dressing room to change into my gown.

Let me tell you, this garment requires a medical degree to assemble. It was a jigsaw puzzle of snaps. I was sweating picturing everyone on the other side of the door wondering what was taking so long. I walked out of the room with the snaps down the front instead of the sides, and it was immediately clear that I had not gone to hospital-gown school. The nurse kindly snapped up a new one for me to change into.

I also didn't get the memo that you're supposed to wait in your dressing room until they come to get you. I figured if I had been called back and was dressed and ready, it was my turn. Definitely not the case. I walked out of my dressing room again and, with everything snapped correctly this time, confidently marched right across the hallway and into the radiation room. I completely missed the gigantic red stop sign with the words DO NOT ENTER. When I walked in, you can imagine my surprise when there was a man in there putting his pants back on. But here I was, waltzing through the huge metal doors and walking in on this semi-naked gentleman.

The nurse raced after me, shouting, "No, no, no!"

She took me by the shoulders and turned me around to exit the room. It turns out, you are *not* supposed to open any doors without explicit permission and a chaperone. So, a note to everyone: Don't walk into a radiation room with a big stop sign on the door. Wait in the dressing room until they ask you to follow them. Then, and only then, can you walk across the hall.

The other step I hadn't completed was stopping at a little office next to the radiation room, where I had to give the nurse my date of birth and confirm I was indeed the patient who was going to receive the radiation treatment. After that, there was a nurse to walk me into the specific room where I would receive my treatment.

Once I was finally in the radiation room, I found it incredibly intimidating. The machine looked like something out of a science fiction film—humongous and futuristic. I could instantly see why there weren't a bunch of these lying around. I supposed I could have googled images of the machine before I got there, but I didn't, and I was properly surprised upon seeing it for the first time.

There was a metal bed in the middle, and it looked like the machine rotated around you. John and my mother had seen everything regarding my treatment until now, and I resisted the urge to take photos to show them what it looked like because I thought this one might freak them out.

On the other side of the room, there were shelves with a ton of eerie-looking face casts. I asked about them and was reminded that cancer can exist all over the body, and those were for patients with brain tumors. The ghostly masks did not ease my mind.

I climbed up on the table awkwardly, not knowing how to position myself. It turns out that was the least awkward part of what followed. Once on the table, I had to unsnap my gown to expose my breast to the male nurse I had met thirty seconds earlier, under lights brighter than the surface of the sun. I kept thinking about how I had one breast deflated and the other out for the nursing staff to see. Modesty has no place in breast cancer.

That's another difference between radiation and chemo. Outside of radiation, you get your breasts examined only by your doctors, whom you know and trust. During each surgery, I was out, thank goodness, while completely uncovered. But on the radiation table, I was embarrassed to be on display. You're exposed in more ways than one because they must position you just so on the bed. For my situation, they also had to prop my arm over my head to ensure the beams targeted the exact right areas. The bed is then adjusted until you are in the precise—and I mean to-the-millimeter precise—location needed.

I was so tense in my first session, just clenched all over. For some reason that I didn't quite understand, I was experiencing more and more anxiety in that moment than I had with anything else up to that point, including pre-op for my double mastectomy. I don't know what it was, but there was something about that room that made me feel vulnerable. It hit me in a totally different way than chemo had. I can't quite put it into words, but in that moment, I deeply felt my cancer. Somehow I was a cancer patient in a different way. I found myself teary-eyed just thinking about the magnitude of it all.

The first session was scary mainly because I didn't know what to expect moment to moment. I had been given a lot of information about what I might experience as a *result* of radiation, but no one had mentioned what it would actually be like to receive it.

The machine rotated around me and I kept my eyes closed because I could only take one thing at a time. I heard the beams go off, and then the machine would rotate with more beams and so on, until I heard over the loudspeaker, "All done. You can move your arm now."

In the sessions to come, I would start to speak the machine's language and to recognize, *Okay, I'm going to be done after this one*. It moves, it clicks. It moves, it clicks. Sometimes, they had to start taking images before they could start the actual radiation, so I'd hear and interpret those clicks too. I became a click-master who could teach a click class.

Of course, I had none of this knowledge for my first round, so I just anxiously kept wondering what was going to happen next. It was like the first time you take a long trip somewhere and it seems to take forever, but your return trip goes by much more quickly because you know what to expect and recognize the markers.

The thing that remained a constant in my mind was how physically exposed I was to radioactivity. Even at the dentist they give you a lead vest. Here, I was naked. The nurses would get me situated just so on the table, make sure my breast was out and my arm was up—and then they would leave the room and go into a safe booth where they wouldn't be in danger of the treatment I was about to receive. I thought about that a lot. They couldn't even be in the same room, and here I was *inside the machine* with no protection, just getting radiated willy-nilly.

The feeling was similar to my chemo sessions, when I had watched my nurse starting my infusions in full hazmat gear while I sat there in sweats watching the drugs go into my veins. This time, the hazmat suit wasn't even enough. There needed to be a wall and window between us. Definitely not the most reassuring situation.

Because my radiation plan was scheduled for five days a week, the rigor of the treatment was mentally taxing. You wake up nearly every day thinking about receiving radiation, and all the other things in your life that simply needed to orbit around your daily trip to the hospital for cancer treatment.

During the day-to-day, it's hard to plan things like work commitments or parent-teacher conferences. I was fully back to work at this point, and it was stressful to make all my daily appointments, calls, and Zooms happen as planned. My schedule was constantly being reworked because the one thing that I could not control was my radiation appointment. For the duration, it means you can't plan a trip beyond a weekend. My brother was getting married during my last week of radiation, and it was a question mark when I would be able to arrive. Ahead of every obligation, you must consider your radiation schedule every day, without fail.

Another thing that was news to me: Your radiation time can change every day. You have an appointment scheduled, but that doesn't mean that time is locked. Things can slow down or speed up, so you are essentially on call. It's all fluid. You have to make it work to continue the course of daily treatment, no matter how difficult.

I once asked one of the nurses, "What happens if you're a school-teacher, or if you're a waiter at a restaurant? What if you don't have the ability to drop everything and leave?"

The radiation team acknowledged that it was a tough situation, but that people receiving treatment had to show up for their daily appointments regardless. The hospital staff was willing to talk to someone's employer to explain the situation, but at the end of the day, there wasn't another option. This was simply the way it worked, and everyone had to get on board.

So many factors contribute to the shifting of radiation schedules. Radiation happens all day, every day. And unlike chemo, for which there are a lot of treatment bays, for radiation there are only a couple of machines. God only knows what these things cost, because they are giant Star Wars space stations taking up the entire room.

I had to mentally wrap my head around how all-consuming it was going to be, how my schedule could change at a moment's notice when they called me with a new time. Sometimes it wasn't even a call that alerted me. I would just get an app notification on my phone that I was now scheduled at a different time. I wanted to write the notification back to say, "Dear App, And what if that time doesn't work?! Can I get some options?"

Every time I opened the app, I did so with trepidation. My work schedule and life schedule were pretty carefully planned out with appointments, work commitments, mom duties. The app did not care. This took some getting used to.

It's not that I don't understand the variety of reasons the times are in flux day in and day out. For instance, there are a lot of people with different health circumstances and different needs that are rightly prioritized. Some are at higher risk and need to come at a different time of day when it isn't as busy. Every case is unique and might require accommodations. Remember, there are only a couple of flying space stations that can deliver treatment, so if one is taken up by another patient, the other appointments have to shift. But it does cause chaos.

As my scheduled appointment times routinely blew out the window and new times were given, I became accustomed to the lack of a schedule. I had to leave lunches before food was served; I had to leave work before we were finished with a meeting. I was told from the beginning (because of course I asked) that it's possible to miss one appointment, but no more. Radiation rounds need to be delivered consecutively without pausing or skipping; delaying an appointment by even a day wasn't feasible.

The funny thing about that, though, was the *hospital* would occasionally have to miss a day because of a holiday closure. So cancer treatment could wait for Thanksgiving weekend or the Fourth of July, but if I had a wedding to go to, that was not going to happen. I understood the logic: We had to stay as close to the schedule as possible because planned holidays or unplanned activities were going to occur.

After a couple of days of radiation, I got into a routine. I knew where to park. Then I headed down to the basement, navigated the hallway maze, checked in, and waited my turn. I never figured out how to snap my gown, though. But I was getting the hang of it. I even started to think, *This is okay. It's just twenty minutes every day for six weeks. I can manage it.*

And that's when I got COVID.

One Thing

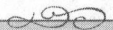

I found it tremendously helpful to make countdowns and lists throughout my treatment. I might be biased given my career in organizing, but it was comforting to be able to cross things off and check boxes. I'm not much of a paper person, so I kept a mental countdown for all my sessions, and I had multiple lists in my Notes app: products to try, things to remember to bring, questions for my doctor—many of which I've shared throughout this book.

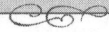

CHAPTER TWENTY-TWO

Nights at the Radiation Basement

R adiation was interacting with my body in very different ways than I had experienced with chemotherapy. I was a new kind of tired. My energy was being zapped, and there was no break in between. Five days a week you get punched, and there isn't much time to recover before it happens again.

So when I felt under the weather one night, I imagined it was just my fatigue ramping up. After all, I knew these treatments built up in your system cumulatively. So it made sense to feel things more acutely as the days went on. But I felt lethargic, not just tired. And then I coughed. My mother and John looked at each other and suggested that I take a COVID test. I humored them and swabbed my nose, then went to my porch chair while I waited. John sat opposite me with the test in front of him, willing it to be negative.

It was positive. Test results *really* were not breaking my way in 2022. I could not catch a break. It's a good thing I was already outside because I immediately became patient zero in the house. John put on a mask, my mother packed a bag to move to a hotel, and the kids were instructed to avoid being in the same room with me.

My head started swimming, thinking about how my body would process this virus, and how this would logistically affect my radiation treatment. I wasn't supposed to miss even one day, so I had no idea how I would navigate this. I called Dr. Kurtz immediately and said, "What in the world do I do?" I was spiraling.

Methodical as always, she jumped into action to call in prescriptions and made sure I had every tool at my disposal. She could take care of my COVID symptoms, but my radiation oncologist, Dr. Chakravarthy, would have to advise us on how to handle the treatment going forward.

When I got in touch with her, I explained that I had just tested positive.

Much to my shock, she said, "We can still treat you while you have COVID." She went on to explain that there would be different protocols, but a nurse would call me to discuss those in the morning.

I don't know what I thought "different protocols" meant, but I didn't expect it to include my radiation appointments moving to the dead of night. That's right, my daily sessions had to be at the very end of the day, when everyone was gone. They couldn't risk me infecting anyone else because so many of us were immunocompromised. So the nursing staff needed time to deeply sanitize the machine after I used it.

There were other protocols in place as well. I would arrive in the passenger pickup section of the hospital, park my car there, and call the nursing desk to tell them I had arrived. One of the nurses would come and get me in—you guessed it—a hazmat suit. They covered every inch of their body, from head to toe. I felt like I had a scarlet letter on my chest as I followed her through the basement and into the radiation room. The maze of hallways felt very different with no other people around.

I could not have imagined that radiation in a dungeon could get *more* depressing. A lot more depressing. It wasn't exactly a social hour before, but now the lights were dim, and I was the only one there. It was seven p.m., and I just wanted to be home with my family. I was forty years old . . . seven p.m. might as well have been midnight. Leaving the comfort of my house alone at such a late hour felt merciless. Until I got COVID, I had always had John or my mom (or both!) during my treatments and doctor visits. I didn't like this new development one bit.

I was already feeling incredibly emotional, and this was putting me over the edge. I just hoped I tested negative soon because I didn't think I could continue that daily dark dungeon march.

The one upside about being a pariah is that you have a lot of time to devote to work. We at The Home Edit were finishing our third book and were in our final rounds of edits. Not being able to do anything or see anyone really increased my productivity. I could crank through chapters pretty quickly. I didn't even have radiation during the day to disrupt my train of thought. I was a captive contributor without distractions.

Eventually, some days later, I tested negative for COVID. Hallelujah! I was very excited to get out of COVID solitary confinement and back into the general population. Radiation was going to go back to just being moderately terrible. I couldn't pick up the phone fast enough to tell the hospital the good news. But it didn't land the way I had expected.

There were still protocols in place at the hospital that hadn't changed since earlier in the pandemic, and we had to follow them even if they didn't align with COVID rules elsewhere. I had tested negative and had no symptoms, but I still had to stay in COVID containment for the next three weeks.

Three more weeks? That felt like a lifetime. Three weeks meant I wouldn't go back to a regular treatment schedule until my last week of radiation. I was so desperate that I actually tried to bargain with the nurse who delivered the news. As though she was going to break long-standing hospital protocol because I was making a persuasive argument.

So off we went five nights a week (once I was negative, at least my mother or John could drive me). We would park in the same spot I'd been using, and I'd call the nurse to let them know I had arrived. Then I'd follow them down to the basement and through the corridors. I felt bad that the poor nurses still, even though I did not have COVID anymore, had to get in the hazmat suit to come get me.

"Just so you know, I don't have COVID anymore," I said to the nurse decked out like an astronaut.

She nodded. "I know, but until the rules change, we still have to treat you like you do."

I don't know why I kept thinking that maybe one night the response would change. I really needed to give it up and just accept things for what they were. You would think too that having the nighttime appointments would mean I didn't have to keep rearranging my schedule, but it actually got worse. Having the last appointment of the day meant every problem, delay, or other contributing factor would push my scheduled time later and later. And in some instances, there would be a cancellation, or they finished earlier, and I would have to drop everything and rush over to the hospital. Sometimes I would go in at 7 p.m., sometimes it would be 4 p.m., and sometimes it would be a random 6:20 p.m. I gave up trying to guess and just kept checking the app for my appointment time.

Being COVID-free didn't help with my radiation schedule, but it did mean I could get back to work in person.

Joanna and I had just launched our podcast, *Best Friend Energy*, and we were recording multiple times a week. During radiation, it's hard to schedule a nail appointment, much less a recording session with a celebrity guest. There were many times I had to run out of the recording to make my radiation time. I kept reminding myself that this would end soon, but it was a very chaotic time for me and my team alike.

I was learning how to go with the flow to the best of my ability, but some days were harder than others. One of the most depressing ones was Halloween. I just wanted to take the kids trick-or-treating and enjoy myself, but my upcoming treatment was looming. I was walking around the neighborhood close to their school when my appointment time was confirmed for the day.

Stella was a cowgirl, but if you know anything about Nashville, she looked like she was part of a bachelorette party because she and her friends were in all pink and sequins. Sutton was Groot from *Guardians of the Galaxy*, which I had never heard of before, but he seemed very excited.

I walked with John, my mom, and the kids while counting down until I had to leave. Then it started to rain and I remember thinking, *This is officially the worst Halloween of all time*. We ducked into a friend's house to let the rain pass before the kids went back out, and before my mom and I had to leave for my radiation appointment. The rain was very symbolic of my mood.

At six o'clock, I hugged the kids goodbye and left them with John to continue trick-or-treating, while I headed to the hospital to get radiation, where there was zero candy. I didn't cry, but I was so, so sad. It had been a long year. I was exhausted from having treatment every day. I was exhausted from being sick all the time and being too ill to fully participate in my life. I was *over* cancer.

Radiation made me feel, more than any other time in my cancer journey, like I couldn't have a minute to myself. There was no grace period at this point, no reprieve. I was a cancer patient through and through, and nothing else.

One Thing

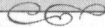

Don't contract COVID during radiation. Do not recommend.

CHAPTER TWENTY-THREE

"Meet Me at Midnight"

Every single day, my north star was November 22. That would be the last day of treatment and I was laser-focused on getting there. With every low moment, at least there was the passage of time, and every day I inched closer and closer to November 22.

One of the great gifts to me in this time was Taylor Swift's *Midnights*, which came out in October. I listened to it nonstop. Every night driving to the hospital, my mother and I would listen to it straight through, which is the exact time it took us round trip. There's a lot on that album that resonated deeply with me. For starters, the album documents thirteen sleepless nights, and I hadn't slept in months. So, lines about being up in the middle of the night hit home in a very big way. Up at night, unable to sleep, I found that listening to these songs brought me real comfort.

Another highlight came mid-November. I was being honored by the American Cancer Society at their annual ball, and I was going to be there come hell or high water. I wasn't quite sure how it was going to work logistically, but I was committed to trying. The evening of the event, I went to radiation as usual, and I brought my gala gown with me. After treatment, I went into my usual dressing room, took off my hospital gown, and put on my gala gown. I walked down the same maze of hallways and went up in the same elevator, but this time I was headed to a black-tie event instead of home.

The event was a fundraiser for the American Cancer Society's Hope Lodge program, which provides free lodging for cancer patients and their relatives while undergoing treatment. It was not lost on me how lucky I was to live in such close proximity to my hospital. So, in the spirit of fundraising for this incredible cause, I let everyone in the room know what I was currently experiencing compared with those who need assistance.

"Two hours ago, I was receiving radiation treatment," I said. "And I was able to get from my house to the hospital, and to this gala, because I'm fortunate enough to live so close to where I receive care."

A very common question you get asked when you show up for chemo or radiation is "Where did you come in from?" Most people receiving treatment do not live fifteen minutes from a world-class hospital. Patients often travel great distances, commute to and from appointments, stay with relatives, or find local housing. I heard the conversations around me every single time I checked in for my own appointments or sat in a waiting room.

Being sick is hard enough. The weekly and daily grind of treatment adds a completely different mental and physical toll. And layering on the difficulty of not living close to your treatment facility feels like an unfair burden. So, it was a good night with a lot of money raised. I hadn't had a good night in a very long time.

Every day was Groundhog Day, just with changing appointment times. I was almost out of COVID confinement, still crossing off the days as they went by. I started to know all the nurses by name and masked face, and could almost (but still not quite) snap my gown by myself. The one thing I noticed, though, with each passing day, was that I was getting so, so very fatigued, and my burn was deepening. I needed this to end.

Finally, November 22 arrived. The day I had been looking forward to since my initial diagnosis. I had a bounce in my step going into radiation. John always waited in the car during treatment because, unlike with chemo, no one is allowed in the room with you. This time, however, he brought his camera and sat in the little waiting room. We hadn't expected the last day of chemo to come so suddenly, without warning, but we knew this was the last day of radiation, and he wanted to document it. It was actually thrilling to be able to walk the same hallways knowing that it was my last day. I had been crawling and scraping my way to the finish line this entire time. And now that I had reached the end, it was very emotional.

Before I went in for my final session, I asked if John could be allowed into the radiation room once I was done. I wanted him to see what it looked like and what I'd been experiencing for all those weeks. He knew so much about my chemo experience and nothing of my radiation experience, so it was important to me. Most people don't see a radiation room unless they're a patient or they march into the room unknowingly.

The second my final radiation treatment ended, the machine shut down and the nurse said into the speaker, "You can put your arm down now." Then they lowered the table and came back in the room to help me up. The floodgates opened before the nurses even entered.

"Oh my God," I said between sobs. "I am done. I am done!"

I could barely see John enter the room through my tears, but he rushed over to me, and we hugged like we had never hugged before. Maybe this was actually over. I didn't even dare to believe it.

I went back to the dressing room to change and laughed when I unsnapped that damn hospital gown for the last time. It was hard to get dressed because I was trembling the entire time, but I managed to get my jeans on. When I rang the bell for chemo I was in my pajamas; I was not going to be caught in anything other than a structured pant this time.

As I exited the dressing room, I came out to a hall lined with my radiation nurses, whom I had come to love. They handed me my brand-new certificate of completion; I had graduated from another phase of cancer treatment. I couldn't contain my tears as I rang the bell three times. Breast cancer wasn't behind me, but this part of my life was. My last stop before leaving was my radiation oncologist.

I hadn't stopped crying yet, and Dr. Chakravarthy remarked, "Usually this is a happy day!"

I explained that it was indeed a very happy day, but also such an emotional one. I had been pushing and pushing to get to the end, and now that I was here, I felt like an ultramarathoner collapsed on the ground after crossing the finish line, trying to catch my breath.

My doctor went through care instructions for the next couple of weeks because my burn would continue to intensify during that window, and we booked our upcoming follow-up appointments.

When she asked if I had any questions, I blurted out the elephant in the room: "Do I have cancer anymore?"

"I can tell you that you have no evidence of disease," she said.

NED, as it's called, was as good as it was going to get. There could be no promises made about tomorrow, and no official proclamations of today, but I was going to wear it like a cancer-free badge of honor.

We decided to have a family dinner to celebrate the end of a very long chapter for all of us. From March 8, when I was diagnosed, to April 8, when I had my double mastectomy and was told the cancer had spread, and through all the subsequent months that followed, it was *finally* November 22. We were going to enjoy this day as much as humanly possible because we had all worked hard to get to this point. Cancer turned out to be a team sport in my household, and the very least we could do was share some dessert.

For the next couple of days, I would wake up and say, "I don't have cancer." I figured if I said it enough times, I would start to actually believe it. People congratulated me, and I would respond with hugs, big smiles, and thank-you messages. So why was I not as happy as I should have been? Why did I have a feeling of dread when someone congratulated me for being done? I realized that my relationship with cancer, once again, was very complicated.

For starters, I recognized that I was not, in fact, *done*. With my primary treatment, yes, but my adjunct treatment (or adjuvant therapy)—additional treatment given to help prevent cancer from reoccurring—would be starting soon. This would consist of two different oral medications—one that I would need to take twice a day—and monthly infusions to shut down my hormone production. My cancer was hormone positive, so I had to reduce my risk as much as possible to prevent reoccurrence. This would be my treatment plan for the next *ten years*.

I was so grateful to everyone who reached out and wished me well, but every time I heard, "It's finally over!" I would think, *It's not and it never will be.*

I also recognized that I had channeled all my emotions and feelings for nearly a year into fighting cancer daily. Now that I no longer had that purpose, I felt lost, like I was drifting in some middle space that didn't have an end. I didn't remember my life before having cancer, and there was no turning back to that life, even with my primary treatment complete. So if I couldn't go back, and I didn't know how to go forward, where did that leave me? I think I assumed that when I rang the final bell, a switch would flip and the clouds would lift. If only it were that easy.

Then the doubt started to creep in. *I only did six rounds of Taxol instead of twelve. What if I did seven weeks of radiation instead of six? Would I feel "done" then? How does everyone know I really received enough treatment?*

I had to continue to remind myself, *There is no evidence of disease.* Whether I had received more treatment or less, there were no guarantees about the future. All I could do was focus on the day in front of me, just as I had done every day prior.

The high of completing treatment was officially over. It was time to figure out how to navigate the present.

One Thing

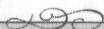

Finishing treatment is very emotional on all levels. In my case, I believed the switch would flip immediately following my last session, and that I would skip out of the hospital and into the sunset. But that didn't happen, and the subsequent days for me were unexpectedly hard. I wish I had known that it's okay—and completely normal—to have a multitude of feelings during this time.

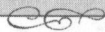

CHAPTER TWENTY-FOUR

The Nameless Sorrow

As November rolled into December, I was starting to struggle. My emotions were all over the place, my fatigue was at an all-time high, and my radiation burn was raging. Great timing for all this because we were flying to Los Angeles for my brother's wedding. All through treatment I had been stressed that my radiation schedule might prevent me from being there that weekend in its entirety. I had been bracing myself to fly in the morning of the wedding, and then immediately back to Nashville. So at least I could cross that concern off my list. But for some reason, I just couldn't get into a celebratory mood.

I didn't know what was wrong with me. This was the actual light at the end of the tunnel that I had been staring at for months! My brother's wedding was meant to be the first moment of pure joy all year. Our first trip as a family in which we didn't have to worry about me landing in the ER or rushing back for chemo. Maybe it was me realizing that I couldn't just pick up where I had left off before my diagnosis and return to my old life. Or that I still couldn't do a single thing without being reminded of my ongoing condition. But I was getting extremely frustrated that I couldn't snap out of it.

Then there were reminders that were impossible to ignore. The dress that I had selected for the wedding had been hanging in my closet, ready and waiting, for a long time. The only problem was that when I had tried it on, my breast expanders were deflated for radiation. Before leaving for Los Angeles, I had refilled my expanders to look as decent as possible in my outfit. But I didn't consider that my expanders would change the fit of the dress. When I went to put the dress on before the wedding, the zipper broke when I tried to zip up the back.

To say I was horrified would be putting it mildly. Frantically, I called the front desk to see if there was a seamstress, or a sewing kit, or tape and glue. I was walking down the aisle, and I really didn't want to be in jeans. The hotel sent someone to help, but try as they might, they could not sew the dress back up. The only solution was to safety-pin the entire back together so it wasn't gaping open. Thankfully, the dress had a capelet that hid the broken zipper and safety pins, but any wrong movement and it would be noticeable. I silently cursed my body for doing this to me and went off to watch my brother and his beautiful bride get married.

Later in the evening, during the reception, my body and dress were having another argument. Under the capelet, the dress was sleeveless. And as warned, my radiation burn had been intensifying following my last session. Where the dress met my armpit was now tearing my skin and causing it to bleed. I tried to ignore it, but pretty soon I had tears in my eyes due to the pain. My mother and Joanna rushed me to my mom's hotel room to change into another dress for the remainder of the evening. I was no longer silently cursing my body; I was loudly enraged with it.

When the wedding was over and I was in my hotel room, I sobbed and sobbed. I wondered if I would ever have a normal day again, a day without trauma, humiliation, pain, or discomfort.

December was a packed month for events, holidays, and travel— which, after so many months of none of those things, was my dream come true. I knew all these things equaled me being happy, but once again, I couldn't access that happy feeling.

Case in point: Joanna and I had been invited to the White House holiday party in D.C. (no big deal) and we were able to bring our husbands with us too. I'd been to the White House during the holidays before (this is my only flex and I stand by it), and let me tell you, there is *nothing* more beautiful. Each room is filled with Christmas in every corner. They must have a tree farm next to the rose garden because there were more than you could possibly count.

Nothing, and I mean nothing, makes me happier than Christmastime. We were staying in Georgetown, which is right out of a Charles Dickens novel. There were wreaths on every lamppost, twinkling lights lining the streets, Christmas carols being sung on the sidewalks; it was pure heaven. We even ate at Le Diplomate, my favorite restaurant. It's perfect year-round, but at Christmas, it's like eating in a magical snow globe. Clearly, I am a Christmas superfan (and yes, we celebrate Hanukkah too).

And yet on that trip, I didn't experience the warm and fuzzy holiday joy in the way I usually would, which was disconcerting. If I was having a hard time in D.C. during *Christmas*, at the White

House holiday party, while being cancer-free, I knew I should be worried.

Perhaps most unlike me, I was having a hard time getting out of bed. Yes, I was tired, but this was something totally different. I stayed in my hotel room with the curtains closed until the very last minute I had to get up and do something. Under normal circumstances, I would be excited to walk around, have lunch, do some shopping . . . but I just couldn't seem to face the day.

It felt like everyone around me had crossed cancer off the list as complete, but I still walked around all day as a cancer patient. It was a lonely feeling because I had a hard time articulating my feelings to those close to me, and I felt guilty mentioning anything to people who checked in. Everyone had been there for me during cancer treatment, and it didn't feel right to burden them further. I also felt guilty talking about it to the general public, who had been rooting for me so consistently. I felt like I was letting everyone down.

And then I realized I had felt this way before. It was right after Stella was born. My friends and family seemed filled with endless joy, whereas I felt like I was looking through a window at them. Having a child was supposed to be the happiest moment of my life. Why wasn't it?

Of course, there was no way I could vocalize my feelings to anyone at the time. They were all over the moon, and I'd be a monster if I told them how I was feeling. I chalked it up to being exhausted and anxious, and I assumed it would pass. But it didn't. I was moody all the time and would spontaneously burst into tears.

Finally, one night, when Stella was three weeks old, nothing was making her go to sleep. I had tried feeding her, giving her a pacifier, bouncing her, walking with her—nothing. I put her down in the crib, hoping she was worn out, but a minute later the crying started again. John went to go pick her back up from the crib, and I shouted, "You always take her side!" At which point we thought, *Okaaaaaay, maybe it's time to call the doctor.* My doctor at the time put me on medication to help ease my depressed feelings, and the clouds lifted shortly after.

But no one had ever said anything about getting post-cancer depression! That would be insane. I had to keep pushing through; this would resolve itself soon.

After D.C. we headed back to California to see our families. The first stop was my parents' house, and then we would move to John's parents' house after. My parents had just moved, so instead of staying with them, we stayed at a beautiful hotel nearby. We hung out with my family during the day doing fun holiday things, and spent the evenings watching Christmas movies with the kids. What could be more perfect? But the depression continued, and my discomfort kept rising.

I had to cut this out *now.* My kids had been through enough—couldn't I at least be happy and in good spirits for them? They'd put on a brave face so many times for my benefit. My mother, John, Sutton, and Stella had sat by my side through it all. They deserved better than this. I knew I needed to try—and I did, but everything continued to feel dull, like the pilot light had gone out. All I could think was, *Am I broken for good? Is this something that I can change or is this my new normal? Is this going to be the way I feel forever?*

I went back to the lesson I had learned a hundred times at this point: If you feel something, say something. So, I called my doctors to tell them what was going on. I was embarrassed to admit any of this to them. They had fought to save my life, and I was about to tell them I was sad? It felt ungrateful, to put it mildly.

But it turned out I *wasn't* alone in having these feelings, and that depression after treatment happens all the time, for a variety of reasons. My psychiatrist recommended that I try a different anxiety medication that targeted more of what I was feeling. It would take a few weeks to kick in, but I could start it right away. The other prescription: I had to do some form of physical exercise. Even if I was tired, I had to push myself to get outside and take a walk. Nothing was going to be effective if I was sleeping all day in a dark room.

I went back to my roots of coming up with solutions and a solid plan. I had a therapy tool kit, a plan for movement, and a plan for medication. I could do this. I had done very hard things already, and getting my mind back on track was going to be one of them.

From California, we traveled to Hawaii for the week leading up to New Year's. This was the trip I had booked right after my fourth round of AC, when I finally felt like I was on the other side of the mountain. I had felt so much hope the day I booked this trip, thinking about the euphoria I would feel to be cancer-free in Hawaii with my family. What on earth could be better?

But now Hawaii felt like a mental test that made me nervous. If I couldn't feel peace and happiness there, of all places, I might have a problem nothing could solve.

Hawaii has always been the most peaceful place for me. When I was younger, my family tried to go once a year for Christmas, so it has always been my happy spot. Which is why it was the obvious place to celebrate the completion of my primary treatment.

We had finally made it to the very spot I had been dreaming about, and as I was sitting in beautiful chaise longues and looking out at the ocean and the pool, I was physically there, but my mind was not.

I'd been so positive during all my treatments, especially about the fact that I was *absolutely* going to make it through to the other side. I'd had a tangible goal then. Now I didn't have anything to really latch on to. I didn't have a finish line, or a completion date, or milestones to mark. All I was left with was anxiety about cancer coming back, and continued treatment for the next decade. I didn't know that I was going to experience grief after beating cancer. I thought I'd be sad only if I lost.

What I started to realize during this time was that my overall healing process might take longer than I thought. Instead of unsuccessfully leaning into the feeling of being "done," I needed to give myself the space to understand I was actually just starting a new phase of my cancer journey. And this phase was just as valid as the last.

One Thing

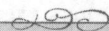

I hope that no one experiences feelings similar to mine following treatment, but if you do, you're not alone. I wish I hadn't kept those early feelings to myself because I could have asked for help sooner. And I wouldn't have wasted over a month beating myself up for not being as happy as I thought I should have been.

Here are some things I found helpful:

- Say it out loud. You might not be ready to share your feelings of depression with others, but you need to be able to admit them to yourself. For me, saying the words out loud made them true and believable. Something I could attack—much like I did with my diagnosis.

- Talk to your doctors. I found over and over again that it never fails. They will figure out a way to help or line up resources. It takes a team to get through cancer and recovery, so don't be afraid to reach out to everyone in your arsenal.

- Talk to your friends. Especially your network of cancer friends. I felt I couldn't find a way to voice my feelings of depression to most of my friends and family, but with my breast cancer friends, I felt safe enough to ask for validation of my feelings and advice for how to process moving forward.

- Physical movement. All my doctors reminded me (and still do) about the importance of physical exercise. My surgeon went as far as to say it was actually a part of my treatment. My psychiatrist said if he could bottle up one thing to help my mental state, it would be exercise. I incorporated thirty minutes of intentional movement every day and it helped tremendously.

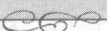

CHAPTER TWENTY-FIVE

New Year, New Drugs

In January I began to see what life was going to look like in the post–primary treatment phase. I was moving into the next phase, known as adjunct therapy or hormone therapy. There are a variety of therapies and drugs available, but in my case, my oncologist and I settled on oral aromatase inhibitors combined with ovary suppression injections.

The differences and distinctions between the various treatment options are well above my level of schooling, but what I understood for certain is that I was hormone positive and had to take every step possible to shut down my hormone production. If this combination of treatments was going to help me do that, I was very much on board.

Remember, being hormone positive allows you options for ongoing treatment, while hormone-negative patients have fewer safety nets. There is no point in shutting down hormone production if you are hormone receptor negative.

This means the paths for hormone-positive and hormone-negative patients eventually diverge. Some of my breast cancer friends who had shared all the same experiences with me suddenly were just done. Not mentally, of course. They had to live with the constant shadow of reoccurring breast cancer more than I did. But physically we were no longer on the same track. We were all back at work, all being full-time parents with full-time schedules, but our day-to-day and week-to-week regimens differed.

As I began this new course of treatment, my doctor told me to monitor my side effects, and if anything became too difficult to manage, we could course correct. My whole life was one big side effect, so I figured a few more wouldn't put me over the top. At least now I had an idea of what things were going to be like. I knew it would likely change or be modified, but at least I had a plan for now.

When I arrived for my first injection, I was taken back to the same rooms where I had received chemo and placed in the same chair. I had *not* been expecting that. Waves of anxiety immediately rolled through me. There was no way I was getting back in that chair. I was never supposed to see that chair again!

It sounded and felt like I was getting shot with a BB gun. It did not feel amazing, but it was bearable. I felt a huge sense of relief. I felt like I could handle that once a month. It was like I was starting to understand the postapocalyptic world that I was in now, and I was actually accepting my new reality. I was even feeling glimmers of happy feelings again. It was a new year and I was moving forward, starting fresh.

I kept reminding myself I needed to give myself time, that this was going to be a process. Except I was in for another rude awakening: Shutting down my hormones drop-kicked me right into menopause.

It happened overnight. My estrogen plummeted and I began having insane hot flashes, gaining weight, having mood swings, and worst of all, I went back to not sleeping. It felt like a bridge too far. I had just experienced so many similar and awful side effects over the past year, and I really was hoping to move on from the worst of them. I had started to take letrozole (my aromatase inhibitor) daily as well, so I imagined the combination put menopause into high gear.

After a couple of months, my doctor wanted to layer on an additional oral medication that was to be taken in the morning and the evening. He told me it was absolutely worth it to further reduce my risk of recurrence. My cancer had proven to be both aggressive and fast-moving, so every single thing I could do to mitigate risk was worthwhile.

But with all the hormone suppressants and medications wreaking havoc on me, I was having a *tough* time. I was perpetually exhausted and could barely leave the house some days. I was just sick *all* the time, both day and night.

This time, I didn't waste more than a couple of weeks before asking for a change in my medication. Every time I had raised the red flag and said, "This is not working for my body," my doctors had been receptive, and we'd found other solutions.

I want to make sure to underscore again and again: *We have to advocate for ourselves.* If I had hesitated to speak up back when I found the lumps in my breast and was declined care by my obgyn . . . I don't even want to consider that outcome. We aren't troublemakers if we say, "There is something wrong here. Can we figure out a solution?"

There have been times in my cancer journey when I realized this right away, and times when I waited too long before speaking up. Hopefully we always arrive at this conclusion sooner rather than later, but the most important thing is that we get there. Not saying anything gets us absolutely nowhere.

After I explained what I had been experiencing, my doctor took me off letrozole entirely and put me on a different aromatase inhibitor called exemestane. My other medication dosage was also adjusted while providing the same benefits. That new combination worked for me. Alas, it didn't get rid of the hot flashes! But it did start to feel like a sustainable solution. And given I would be at this for ten more years, sustainable was the name of the game.

If a perfect medication regimen existed, we would all be on it. But the reality is that we need to make concessions to remain healthy. It's actually a gift that these treatments are available to those of us who are lucky enough to receive them. I often remember something my doctor once told me: We always have to remember that it's the cancer that is the enemy, not the medication. The medication, even with the side effects that come along with it, is there to save our lives. It took me a long time to achieve this realization, but I feel some peace of mind now that I know I'll be on this treatment plan for the foreseeable future.

I've now graduated to an injection that's every three months at a much larger dose rather than once a month at a smaller dose. It feels the same! But at least I get to have two months off between injections. I also still experience both medication side effects and sustained effects from what my body has suffered. It can be frustrating at times that I'm assumed to be in perfect health at this point when I feel anything but. I'm still fatigued. I have setbacks, I have limitations, I get nauseated, I get sick. And I'm still battling cancer, though in a much more private way. I'm still not feeling 100 percent—yet the world can't see that. To them, I'm a survivor. In truth, I'm still a cancer patient.

One Thing

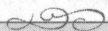

When it comes to adjuvant therapy, there are truly so many options. Most of my hormone-positive friends are on a drug called tamoxifen, but because I travel by plane so much for work, I couldn't chance the higher risk of blood clots. Something as simple as that made me choose aromatase inhibitors instead. It's really important to talk to your doctor and share aspects of your lifestyle that might impact treatment options. And if something isn't working, ask for a different solution; they exist.

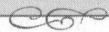

CHAPTER TWENTY-SIX

What and Who Helped,
What and Who Didn't

This has been a *long* journey, and in some ways, it's still just beginning. I find that I have to continue to adapt to my new normal, continue to monitor my side effects, and continue not to put pressure on myself to be the way I was.

For instance, I will never leave the house without Zofran for nausea. It just will never happen. And I continue to lean on some of my most treasured comfort objects: the pajamas I wore during chemo and the blanket I used to stay warm, the silk scarves of my mother's that I wore on my head when I didn't have hair. Those items still make me feel protected, like when I used to take my stuffed animal with me to preschool.

I'm not a believer in holding on to very much. In fact, I've built a whole business based on that philosophy. But in this instance, all these items amount to feeling loved, considered, and cared for. I thought once I was done with chemo I'd want to delicately put these items away and attempt to move on, but I can now respect that they served a purpose and still hold a place in my life. I still use my "Clea Kicks Cancer" bag every time I go for an infusion.

Then there are the people. I'm more bonded than ever to those who were good to me while I was at my sickest. In particular, I had the most amazing support from John, my kids, my mom, and my friends. I am so lucky to be able to say that my inner circle was *that* strong. And I was so thankful for everyone who showed up in any way, whether with food, cards, flowers, or a warm comment on Instagram. This list of people expanded beyond my wildest dreams.

I know my situation is different because I'm a public person, which means in addition to notes from friends and acquaintances, I also received a very sweet get-well card and a knitted hat from a Delta flight attendant. But no matter the scale or the circumstance, compassion will knock you off your feet.

And yet there is a flip side. When you have cancer, you need to focus on your wellness and recovery. And as I continued to progress, there were people who just didn't show up for me. It was, and is, disappointing. But I've learned to leave space for other people's choices, even if they don't align with my expectations.

It's hard to describe this relationship aspect of cancer treatment without sounding selfish. It took me a long time to accept the sad truth that people get illness fatigue. They go through it with you, they give you their well wishes and their love, and then they need to move on. Not everyone is meant to stick with you through the hard stuff, and you *really* recognize those who do. It's a long road and you can't expect everyone to be up for the journey.

Most of the time when people ask me how I'm doing, I don't answer honestly, because no one needs to get into the intricacies of metabolic shifts and night sweats. They want me to say I'm feeling better—great, even!—or at the very least that I am doing pretty well. It's a buzzkill to say, "Yes, I beat cancer. Yes, I have no evidence of disease. But it's still something I think about and deal with on a daily basis." It's natural and normal for people not to understand what it's like at this point because it's bewildering and layered. Realizing that most people around you are doing their best helps you stay focused on what matters.

My goal is to stay cancer-free. That is my first and last thought every single day. I don't necessarily verbalize it to everyone, but it's in my every waking moment. Other things in life fade into the background.

In the aftermath of primary treatment, if, God willing, you have the ability to receive further treatment, you might have to start using your words instead of your thoughts. Even though my journey had ended for most people, I found the need to make the invisible visible. I learned to say, "I need to leave early," "I need to take a nap," "I wish I could be there but I can't overdo it."

Joanna can attest to how foreign these words are for me. I'm always the first person to say yes to a dinner party, and always the last person to leave. My energy tank has always recharged by being out and about doing things, not staying at home watching TV in bed. We don't even have a TV in our bedroom! Taking my fast-paced life down several notches ran counterintuitive to my entire life experience.

There was a funny moment at a work event a few months post-treatment. Joanna and I were there together, and as the time ticked on, she pulled me over to the side of the room to tell me, "I'm really worried about you!" Naturally I assumed she thought I was pushing myself too hard. But instead, she said, "I'm worried you're turning back into your old self!" She had come to enjoy my need to be in bed by nine p.m., and going back to a later bedtime was really not going to work for her.

Lucky for Joanna, the times we've stayed at an event for an extra hour have ended up being few and far between. So, my life for now, and for the foreseeable future, includes periods of rest and the ability to say no. I'm simply not back to the way I was before. My hair might be a little bit longer, but I'm still playing catch-up.

As I've said so many times in this book, cancer is *complicated*. A lot goes into it. Being sick could still provide the most loving and happiest of moments, and healing might cause depression. I didn't know what to expect initially, which is why I wanted to write this book. I want people to at least know from my perspective the ups and downs that I went through. There was so much good in conjunction with the bad; so many moments I thought I could never get through, but I did; lessons I never would have learned; relationships I never would have had.

If the good, the bad, and the ugly can help anyone in this situation, or even those adjacent to someone in this situation, my journey will have been worth it. So many people—husbands, friends, wives, parents, children—need to understand what this side is like, so they know how to be compassionate. Loved ones are empathetic and caring, but no one can be expected to show up in a meaningful way without knowing what's meaningful. I certainly wouldn't have known how until it happened to me.

One Thing

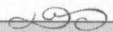

Personally, I have never been great at maintaining boundaries. I'm a people pleaser who says yes to everything and everyone—often to my detriment. During cancer treatment, everyone has pretty reasonable expectations of your limits, but not so much on the other side. Saying no or speaking up can be a challenge for a lot of us, but it's necessary.

I have always been a more-the-merrier, let's-have-another-drink, stay-up-late kind of person. My friends knew they could count on me for dinner and a concert any night of the week. So in this different phase of my life, I had to first accept my new limitations and then accept my necessary boundaries. I had to get comfortable with phrases like "I can't." Which is not something I was used to saying in any part of my life.

During active treatment, it was a given that I couldn't do most things. So as I moved into recovery, I took that same language and attitude and applied it to new situations. Did I love having to turn plans down or leave a party early? No. But I recognized that I must, and everyone around me recognized it as well.

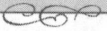

CHAPTER TWENTY-SEVEN

Reconstruction

S urgery feels like a much easier thing to describe than the twists and turns of hormone therapy. And yet I didn't anticipate how twisty and turny the reconstructive process was going to be for me.

I had to wait nearly a year following the end of radiation before I could begin my reconstruction surgery. So if you add that to the eight months I spent before I completed radiation, I had my breast expanders in for a total of one year and eight months. That is quite a long time to have your skin stretched by a device placed behind your breast muscle. It didn't feel great, I'll tell you that. I was counting down the days to kick the expanders to the curb.

I met with my plastic surgeon in advance to discuss my options and potential alternative plans if he needed to pivot.

The first thing he said when he opened up my robe and saw me was, "Wow, Clea, you have been through a lot."

"Thank you for recognizing that," I said, about to burst into tears.

Next, he examined me and told me that I was going to need fat grafting for the area surrounding the implants. He warned me that we'd probably be seeing each other a few times and that this would likely not be my last surgery.

"This isn't going to be the final, this isn't going to be the end," he said.

I would be getting implants plus fat as a swap for my expanders, so I had a bunch of questions about what that would look and feel like. I left the office feeling confident about my upcoming procedure. I wasn't just ready, I was *excited*. There was no love lost between me and my expanders.

Suffice it to say, when I showed up at the hospital bright and early on November 2 for my surgery, I was in the best mood I'd been in since the ordeal had begun. We went through the same process of a bunch of doctors asking me questions, my surgeon drawing on me with a Sharpie, and the painful prick of the IV needle (for me, getting an IV needle in the hand has often been more more painful than the actual procedure), but nothing could diminish my elation over the fact that this was finally happening. As I was wheeled back to the operating room, well, everything went black at that point because the anesthesia kicked in. . . .

I gradually woke up and became vaguely aware of my surroundings. But I was alert enough to ask for various snacks and a Diet Coke. There's something about peanut butter crackers in the recovery room; somehow they are extra-delicious. I was munching away happily when John came back to see me. He said that while it went well, it wasn't as smooth as they had hoped (John has officially reached his quota for delivering bad news in the recovery room).

For starters, my radiated side had an inch and a half of scar tissue to contend with. We always knew radiation would make reconstruction difficult, and here we were. My right breast expander had also sunk into my rib cage—as if I couldn't despise them more. And to top it off, I had lost so much skin during my necrosis surgery that the fold under my right breast was really tight. All this information was given to me while I ate tiny Ritz crackers. Well, it looked like I already had to make an appointment for a follow-up surgery.

While I was trying to take it all in, I went to take a drink from my Diet Coke, but when I picked up the can, my right arm immediately dropped. Well, that was strange. But sometimes when you come out of anesthesia your muscles need a bit to wake up. I figured my arm was just still asleep.

John carefully helped me get dressed and walk to the car. He had a pillow ready to put between me and the seat belt, and a carefully mapped route that didn't include speed bumps. When we got home, I gave my mother and kids air hugs and sat down for dinner. Everyone was staring at me like I was going to collapse any moment, but I really did feel okay sitting at the dining table. It was picking up my fork with my right hand that was causing me the most trouble.

I woke up the next morning feeling like I'd been hit by a truck. I hadn't seen under the bandages yet, but I imagined I looked that way too. Still, this was a *celebratory* surgery. This time, I wasn't marching toward my first round of chemo. This time, I could get better every day without impending dread. I put on my loosest garments and sat drinking coffee with Joanna and my mother in the living room. They still kept eyeing me like I was going to need to be airlifted back to bed, but my pain felt manageable. The only thing that was still bothering me was my arm. I even had to drink my coffee with my left hand.

My surgeon called to check in on me, and I cheerfully told him I was doing great, even though I felt like I had been flattened by a stampede of bulls. I figured it was ridiculous to ask, but if I had learned anything . . .

I explained that my arm was still numb following surgery. I couldn't do normal things with my right hand like apply face cream, hold a cup, pick up a handbag, and so on. Whenever I tried, my arm would just drop straight down with zero control. He confirmed what I had already assumed: This wasn't normal.

Just *great*. Is the universe kidding? Can't I just live? Apparently not, and I had to make an appointment to see an "extremities surgeon."

My arm ended up having nerve damage from the surgery and would just need time to repair itself. It was a good reminder, for the one millionth time, that everything is unpredictable. While I'd thought the only physical therapy I was going to need was for my limited range of motion, now I'd need PT for different muscles in the same arm.

After a few days, I was able to look under the bandages to see my breasts for the first time. I don't know what I was expecting, exactly, but something akin to what a normal boob job looks like. When I looked at myself in the mirror, I was crestfallen. My breasts were still scarred all over and screamed mastectomy. They just felt better. All of my previous surgeries had not set me up for success in the looks department. I had been told I would likely need subsequent surgeries, so maybe this was just a stepping stone to something better.

When Dr. Perdikis first explained this was a multistep process, I assumed that additional surgeries would be strictly for vanity. I

considered myself low maintenance on that front. I'm not an un-
derwear model. My breasts didn't have to be perfect. In my mind,
when I first heard, "This might take a few surgeries," I replied,
"Oh, sir, I don't care what they look like at this point. Anything's
better than what I've had."

The joke was on me, of course. There would be more surgeries
for a variety of reasons, and yes, my need to feel whole when I
looked in the mirror was one of them. I was also going to have to
have my ovaries and fallopian tubes taken at some point (to reduce my risk further), but one thing at a time. I had a lot of healing to do, in more ways than one.

One Thing

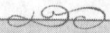

One would think I would be great at no longer having expectations going into a procedure, but I think it's just the human condition to get attached to an outcome. It would have served me, however, to keep an open mind about each part of the process. I think I would have experienced a lot less disappointment if I hadn't been so committed to the expected result.

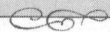

CHAPTER TWENTY-EIGHT

What Comes Next

Overall, things have begun to stabilize. My medication is doing its job, my infusions are still just every three months, and my upcoming surgeries have been scheduled. The hope is that this all equals a cancer-free future.

There will always be days of feeling sick or tired. There will probably be new and different medications, with new and different side effects. But the official checklist that I had, ramping from diagnosis to surgery to chemo to radiation to reconstruction, is complete. Do I feel complete? No. And I probably won't for some time. But I do feel like I'm making significant progress toward that reality. I am grateful to have come this far.

I've become more comfortable with the lack of control that comes with cancer. I feel more stable with instability. I don't believe in blind acceptance—accepting something shitty is not a great way to live—but I think I've learned to accept that I can't control as much as I thought I could. I've also learned that I can adapt to more than I thought I could, that I can recover more easily than I thought I could, and that I can handle more than I thought I could.

With that knowledge and that comfort, I can move forward little by little.

Beating cancer, both physically and mentally, takes *so much* work. You need to steady yourself and stay positive, looking toward the next good thing instead of dwelling on the negative thing in front of you. To this day, whenever my phone rings and it's a doctor's office (which it always is), I stiffen, assuming it's bad news. But sometimes they just want to tell me that my blood panel came back with flying colors. Whatever the scenario, I feel much more prepared to dwell in the unknown.

When I look back at the past couple of years, I see that there were huge challenges and very difficult, intense moments, but there was also so much *goodness.* You'll never experience your own funeral. But this was a moment in my life unlike any other, in which I experienced that deep outpouring of love while I was alive.

The cost was great and the stakes were huge. I was fighting for my life. But when I think about the whole experience, I don't have even the residue of sadness. I felt and feel the love and support. I don't want to go through it again, but what a remarkable thing to have experienced, and what a stronger person I am for having lived through it.

Okay, a Few More Things

Things I Told My Kids:

- This is the plan, but just know that certain things might change, and that's okay.

- You can ask me anything, anytime.

- Is there anyone, like a friend or teacher, you want to tell?

- Is there anything that makes you afraid?

- Cancer might make me look different or feel different, but I am still the same.

Ways to Answer the Question "How Are You Doing?"

- Surviving, not thriving.

- I've had better days.

- I definitely feel the impact.

- I have my ups and downs.

- Grateful to be here.

When People Want to Help, They Can:

- Drive you to an appointment.

- Drop off a meal.

- Host a playdate for the kids.

- Visit the house (I always said I would love company for an hour, but then I would need to rest).

- Take you wig shopping.

Can't-Put-Down Books

- *Throne of Glass* series by Sarah J. Maas

- *The Guest List* by Lucy Foley

- *The Housemaid* by Freida McFadden

- *None of This Is True* by Lisa Jewell

- *The Only One Left* by Riley Sager

Things to Consider to Prepare for Doctor Visits

- Bring a list of questions.

- Have a second person present to take notes. There is a lot to digest in these appointments, and it's hard to take it all in at once.

- Be honest about what you are experiencing so the doctor can best help you.

- Wear a button-down shirt to make breast exams and expander fills easy. I never had to change into a robe!

Things to Eat When Nothing Else Tastes Good

- Saltines

- Ramen

- Matzo ball soup

- Apples
- Pickles
- Ginger chews

Some Good Books About Cancer

- *Not the Breast Year of My Life* by Cara Sapida
- *Crazy Sexy Cancer Tips* by Kris Carr with a foreword by Sheryl Crow
- *If It Makes You Healthy* by Sheryl Crow
- *Hoda: How I Survived War Zones, Bad Hair, Cancer, and Kathie Lee* by Hoda Kotb
- *Beat Breast Cancer like a Boss* by Ali Rogin
- *The Breast Cancer Book* by Val Sampson and Debbie Fenlon

Breast Cancer Organizations to Connect with for More Information

- American Cancer Society (ACS)
- Susan G. Komen
- Breast Cancer Research Foundation (BCRF)
- National Breast Cancer Foundation
- National Comprehensive Cancer Network (NCCN)

Reminder

If you're feeling low at any point, I hope you'll look at this picture my son drew and feel the same boost to your spirits as I do. All of us are tougher than we know.

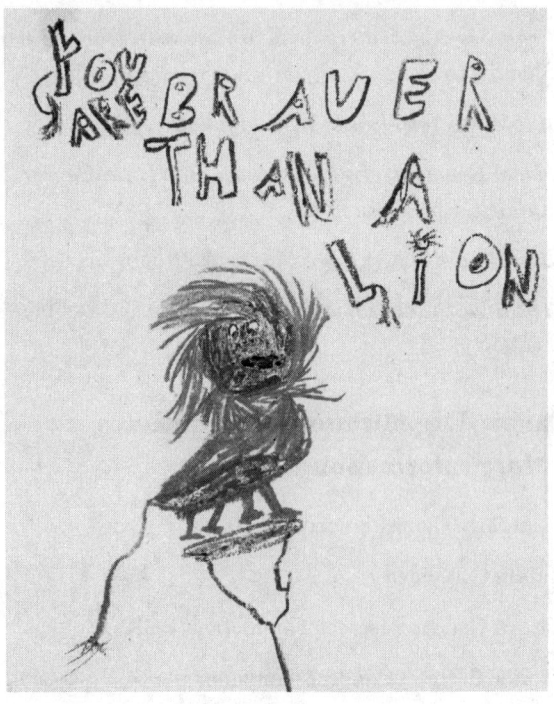

My son, Sutton (age eight), drew me this picture while I was undergoing chemotherapy in the summer of 2022.

Acknowledgments

I want to thank ~

My husband, John, who has never missed a doctor's appointment and has held my hand through this journey. I love you endlessly.

My children, Stella and Sutton, who are stronger and more resilient than I could have imagined. And who sent me off to treatment with a card that said "Don't let chemo make you emo." You both are my reason why.

My mother, who dropped everything in her life to move in with us until I rang the bell on the last day. That time will be forever cherished.

Joanna, who is the best friend anyone could ever have. I am so lucky.

My father, my brother and sister-in-law, and John's family for the endless stream of love. Thank you for being there.

All the friends and family who sat with me when I needed it, checked in on me, and kept me in their prayers.

Dr. Emily Kurtz, Dr. Ben Park, Dr. Ingrid Meszoely, Dr. Galen Perdikis, and Dr. Bapsi Chakravarthy for quite literally saving my life.

My amazing family at The Home Edit and Hello Sunshine. Thank you for working so hard when I could not. Reese, Sarah, and Maureen—I could not have gotten though this without your support.

Maria Shriver for believing that I could write this book.

My agent, Lindsay Edgecombe; my collaborator, Ada Calhoun; my lawyer, Matt Feil; my business managers, Kris Wiatr and team; my manager, Alix Frank; and my adviser on all things, Raina Penchansky. Thank you for being there for me since day one.

The entire team at Penguin Random House, including Isabelle Alexander, Kim Daly, Tess Espinoza, Molly Fessenden, Meg Leder, Rebecca Marsh, Randee Marullo, Shelby Meizlik, Nick Michal, Jason Ramirez, Madeline Rohlin, Kate Stark, Mary Stone, Alexis Sulaimani, Amy Sun, Kym Surridge, Brian Tart, Joan Wong, and Elizabeth Yaffe.